THE JUICE CLEANSE RESET DIET

THE JUICE CLEANSE RESET DIET

7 Days to Transform Your Body for Increased Energy, Glowing Skin, and a Slimmer Waistline

LORI KENYON FARLEY
and **MARRA ST. CLAIR**

TEN SPEED PRESS
Berkeley

Published in the United States by Ten Speed Press, an imprint of the Crown Publishing Group, a division of Random House LLC, a Penguin Random House Company, New York.
www.crownpublishing.com
www.tenspeed.com

Ten Speed Press and the Ten Speed Press colophon are registered trademarks of Random House LLC.

Library of Congress Cataloging-in-Publication Data

Kenyon Farley, Lori, author.
 The juice cleanse reset diet : 7 days to transform your body for increased energy, glowing skin, and a slimmer waistline / Lori Kenyon Farley and Marra St. Clair.
    pages cm
1. Fruit juices—Therapeutic use. 2. Vegetable juices—Therapeutic use. 3. Detoxification (Health) 4. Reducing diets. 5. Reducing exercises. I. St. Clair, Marra, author. II. Title.
 RM237.K46 2014
 613.2—dc23
                          2013035508

Trade Paperback ISBN: 978-1-60774-583-9
eBook ISBN: 978-1-60774-584-6

Printed in the United States of America

Design by Sarah Adelman
Cover photograph by Katie Newburn

10 9 8 7 6 5 4 3 2 1

First Edition

CONTENTS

ACKNOWLEDGMENTS

Our heartfelt gratitude to our dedicated team of wellness warriors at Ritual Wellness: Debbie, Donald, Emil, Jeff, Kaela, Lou, Luis, Markie, Sal, Tyler, and countless others. Without you all, we would not be able to deliver bottles of nutritious freshly pressed organic juice to our clients every day.

To our loyal customers and friends who believed in and supported our vision from the very first day.

To our husbands, Richard Farley and Tom St. Clair, for their patience while we created this book, for allowing themselves to be test cases for new recipes, and for their unyielding faith in our abilities.

To our parents and siblings for always encouraging us to follow our passion for wellness and teaching us that you can accomplish your biggest dreams if you are willing to work hard and you believe you will succeed.

To our agent, Steve Troha, for holding our hands and guiding us skillfully and enjoyably through the process, and to Lindi Stoler for having the vision to see this book even while it was only a tiny seed germinating in our imaginations.

To our brilliant and insightful editor, Julie Bennett, for believing in our project and, more importantly, for helping us organize our thoughts into something you would want to read and be inspired to follow.

To each person reading this book, for taking the first step toward prioritizing your health.

INTRODUCTION
HOW YOU GOT HERE

"The human animal is adapted to, and apparently can thrive on,
an extraordinary range of different diets, but the Western diet,
however you define it, does not seem to be one of them."

—Michael Pollan, *In Defense of Food: An Eater's Manifesto*

Who isn't looking for quick and easy ways to lose weight, look
younger, have more energy, and get healthy? In our constant quest
for improvement, we eat premade processed food, count points, and
drink powdered shakes; we pay for facials, peels, laser treatments,
and fillers; we shoot caffeinated energy drinks; and we get our fat
sucked out, melted down, and sweated away. These quick-fix methods
rarely have lasting results, but we try the latest fads again and again
only to end up disappointed when the programs, products, diets, and
treatments fail to deliver on their promises.

To see results on the outside, you have to focus on improving the
inside. If you're struggling to lose those last five pounds, can't seem
to shake that midafternoon slump, and have started noticing bags
under your eyes, it's time for a reset. By resetting your system, you
create the right internal environment for what you want to accomplish, whether that's increasing your energy level, dropping a few
pounds, reducing your cravings for sugary food, creating glowing

skin, or just plain getting healthy. To get the results you want, you must first clear your body of the toxins and acidity that prevent it from absorbing nutrients.

People ask us all the time, is cleansing really necessary? Aren't our bodies designed to clean themselves through the function of the liver, kidneys, and miles of digestive tract? The short answer is yes. And while it's true that our bodies are able to fight off infections, remove waste from the digestive system, combat diseases, and clean out the toxins we ingest, these days we subject our bodies to a lot of unnatural ingredients, whether by choice or inadvertently, which makes it harder than ever for our bodies to keep up.

THE WONDERS OF FOOD TODAY

Thanks to science and advances in the food industry, there are now pesticides that can keep wildlife from eating our produce before we can pick it. Seeds are genetically engineered to produce fruit that is perfectly shaped, is resistant to diseases, and ripens just when the growers want it to ripen. Inventions like argon gas allow farmers to pick produce before it has ripened, ship it across the country, and spray it so that it reaches the perfect color to appear ripe once it hits the supermarket shelves. Thanks to these shipping practices, you're not limited to the type of fruit grown in your part of the country or the world, but have access to nearly every variety all year long.

Similarly, cows, chickens, and pigs are raised from birth to slaughter in a much shorter time frame than they were fifty years ago. Livestock are fed engineered grain to mature them more quickly, and treated with antibiotics to protect against diseases prevalent in their poor living conditions and caused by the hormones they are injected with. Chickens and pigs are fed fatty diets and their movement is restricted to help them plump faster. Fish are farmed to increase the population of certain breeds, while exposing them to more antibiotics and pesticides than their wild kin.

In an effort to accommodate our quickening lifestyle, grains are processed to speed up preparation time. Rather than cooking steel-cut oatmeal for breakfast, we buy breakfast cereal made from refined white flour. These flours are generally derived from a whole grain. During the milling process, the kernel is put through a high-heat process that removes the germ and bran (which contain 90 percent of the nutritional content of the kernel), leaving only the endosperm (starch). To replace those nutrients lost in processing, artificial vitamins and minerals are sprayed onto the finished cereals or baked goods.

Here's the issue. Real food and manufactured food are not the same things to your body, even if they look the same to a scientist. Nutrients and vitamins and minerals can be created in the lab and glued onto processed food, but our bodies can tell the difference. Even if you start with a nice ripe orange, full of antioxidants and vitamin C, once you juice, heat, and pasteurize it, the nutrients are dead, and the enzymes necessary to help your body absorb the vitamins have been killed off, too. But it'll stay fresh on the grocery store shelves for months on end.

We eat processed, manufactured foods created in a lab or a factory rather than unprocessed foods grown in the ground. Add to that all of the environmental toxins we're exposed to—airplanes crossing the skies emitting exhaust that contains a variety of air pollutants, farming methods that pollute the atmosphere with carbon dioxide at a faster rate than plants can produce oxygen, natural gas extraction methods that release methane into the atmosphere, and manufactured waste that fills our oceans with chemicals—and it's easy to see how the overload is more than our bodies can keep up with!

WE ARE WHAT WE EAT

All of these changes to our diets and the results of new food-production technology are catching up with our bodies. Today, obesity is officially an epidemic. Forty years ago, we fought to end world hunger, yet today we have a greater chance of dying from overnutrition (the health consequence of obesity) than malnutrition. According to the World Health Organization (WHO), worldwide obesity has nearly doubled since 1980, and 65 percent of the world's population live in countries where being overweight or obese kills more people than being underweight does. Our parents wouldn't let us leave the dinner table without cleaning our plates, citing all of the starving children around the world, but if you clean your plate today, you consume twice as much food as you would have because serving sizes have grown to such monstrous proportions.

A few decades ago, pregnant mothers worried mainly about the possibility of their babies being born with low birth weight or Down syndrome. Today, attention-deficit disorder, autism, and asthma are also prevalent. Allergies and sensitivities to gluten, nuts, eggs, dairy, pollen, and so on are all but commonplace. Children suffer in increasing numbers from adult diseases like type 2 diabetes, hypertension, and depression. Medical researchers predict that today's children will be the first generation to die at a younger age than their parents.

We spend more money in the United States on sickness than on wellness. We treat the symptoms and the effects rather than the cause. But by changing what you put into your body, you can take back control over your health. Yes, real food may be a bit pricier than its manufactured substitutes, but in the long run, your body will thank you. The increased energy, wellness, and quality of life you will experience, along with a decrease in doctor's visits, prescription drugs, and days of feeling less than optimal, make the trade-off a relatively easy one.

Health Stats from the World Health Organization

- Nearly 1.6 billion adults worldwide are overweight and 400 million are obese. *Overweight* and *obesity* are defined as abnormal or excessive fat accumulation that may impair one's health. Body mass index (BMI) is commonly used to classify overweight and obesity in adults. It is defined as a person's weight divided by the square of his height. People who have a BMI greater than or equal to 25 are considered overweight; a BMI greater than or equal to 30 is considered obese.

- The United Nations reported that in 2000, the number of people suffering from overnutrition (defined as health-related issues caused by obesity) was over 1 billion; 800 million people suffer from malnutrition.

- The number of children affected by autism has increased in the past forty years from 1 in 10,000 to 1 in 150 in some states.

- Diabetes-related deaths are on track to increase by more than 50 percent in the next ten years. More than 180 million people worldwide currently have type 2 diabetes.

- Worldwide, cancer-related deaths are projected to increase by 45 percent in the next twenty years.

- Heart disease is the number one killer in the United States, with cardiovascular diseases killing more than 17 million people in 2005. Up to 80 percent of premature heart attacks and strokes are preventable with diet and lifestyle changes.

THE PATH TO RITUAL WELLNESS

Many years ago, we were inspired to make dietary changes for ourselves, which started us on our journey to founding Ritual Wellness.

Lori's Story

Having been diagnosed as a teenager with a rare syndrome that prevents my ability to digest animal protein, I developed an interest in diet and wellness. Being a vegetarian in upstate New York definitely made me different, and as an athlete, it was a challenge for me to make sure I was eating the right foods to sufficiently fuel my workouts and enough protein to rebuild muscle teardown. I developed an interest in cooking, experimenting with food, and learning about nutrition as a way to take control over my diet and health.

As a career, however, I pursued a more lucrative path. I got my law degree, became a member of the bar, went to work in finance, and was running a hedge fund by my mid thirties. For the next three years, it was like a fairy tale; the market was booming, and so was my career. I was splitting my time between Newport Beach, California, and New York City. I was training for a fitness competition, working out with a personal trainer five days a week, doing Pilates the other two days, and working ninety hours a week. Four years later, everything had changed. The market fell out from under us and I developed pneumonia. Three rounds of heavy antibiotics cleared the infection but left me as sluggish and lethargic as the winding-down hedge fund. I knew I needed to make a change to regain my health.

Marra, who was my Pilates instructor at the time, suggested juicing, but I found it to be tedious and time-consuming. Although I loved creating new recipes, I didn't enjoy cleaning the juicer! I searched the country, trying to find a cleanse that was organic (without fillers or artificial ingredients) and that had enough nutrients and protein to allow me to continue with my fitness training. It didn't seem such a product existed.

Marra's Story

As a full-time Pilates instructor in Newport Beach, California, I had many clients who were slim and toned, but who did not make their health and nutrition a priority. Lori was one of those clients. I saw how the antibiotics and stress of her job had worn her down, so I suggested she use juice to heal and rebuild herself, because that's what worked for me when I was in a similar state.

While in college, I had been diagnosed with celiac disease. At the time, it was much less common, and not well understood. I lost excessive weight, became malnourished, lacked energy, and constantly struggled with bloating and stomach pain. When I discovered I was allergic to gluten and wheat, I was thrilled to have the answers to heal myself but confused about what to eat. My Italian family was even more confused, since pasta was a staple in my household. I began to study nutrition, especially books promoting healing through diet. I discovered how juicing could repair the damage that gluten had caused to my digestive system and how I could get back on the path toward optimal health by changing my diet.

After an accident left me with a back injury, I began taking Pilates as a method of rehabilitation and strengthening. I obtained my Pilates certification and, after graduating from college, followed my heart to Paris to be part of the team that set up the first Pilates studio there.

When I returned to California, I began my private Pilates and wellness practice, and met Lori when she became a client. When she told me about her difficulties finding a great juice-cleanse product that she could buy instead of make herself, we realized that there was a hole in the market. The idea for Ritual Wellness and the Reset Cleanse was born.

Over the next year, we both obtained our nutrition certifications and began developing formulations that included the best ingredients for cleansing and detoxing while flooding the body with organic nutrients. We tested the recipes on everyone we knew to make sure the juices tasted amazing and people achieved their desired goals of reduced weight, healthier cravings, and increased energy levels.

OUR RESET CLEANSE

Since we founded Ritual Wellness in 2010, we have developed a nationwide client base. We ship fresh, cold-pressed, organic juice cleanses daily to executives, stay-at-home moms, students, actors, athletes, and everyone in between. We've been thrilled by the successes people have experienced on our juicing programs and we're honored that we get to share our passion for health with so many people. Perhaps most rewarding, though, are the amazing testimonials we receive from our customers every day. Whatever their reasons for embarking on the Reset Cleanse, our clients have all experienced similar results. After three days of drinking organic, raw juices, they tell us they feel reset—whether it's their attitude toward food or their energy levels, metabolism, taste buds, cravings, digestive system, weight, or beauty—they feel like they've jump-started their overall health. Many of our customers claim that it's easier for them to make better dietary choices following the cleanse; they feel like they've been set on a healthier life path. They have a newfound zest for life! And anytime they feel themselves slipping back into their old unhealthy habits (which happens to the best of us), they do another Reset Cleanse to get right back on track.

THE JUICE CLEANSE RESET DIET

The Juice Cleanse Reset Diet is the program we developed from all of our research, experience, and first-hand observation. It provides a simple and easy way to help you reset your attitude, energy level, metabolism, taste buds, weight, and beauty. We'll talk more about what it means to reset all of these areas in the next chapter, but generally speaking, this is about producing weight loss and new levels of health, youth, and energy without resorting to quick fixes or invasive procedures.

CHRIS D., OLYMPIC SKIIER • I generally do a Reset Cleanse every time I come home from a major competition. I train hard and push my body to extremes, and when I am taking a break from skiing, the break from eating is just as valuable. Although I normally eat very well, I still find that the massive quantities of nutrients in the juices really rejuvenate and reenergize me.

Recently I had a bad crash in France while skiing in the World Cup. I injured my knee, and had to have surgery to repair it back home in Colorado. The procedure was a success, but between the anti-inflammatories, painkillers, and anesthesia, I felt terrible and sluggish. I really needed my energy high, to rehab and heal quickly. I ordered a three-day Seasonal Reset Cleanse, and was really stoked to find the box on my doorstep two days later. Not only did the juices rid me of the sluggish, hazy feelings, but they also renewed my energy level and my attitude. I am training hard in the gym, my knee is getting stronger every day, and I am confident I will be back on the tour sooner than my doctor predicted. Thank you, Lori and Marra, for creating such an awesome product!

After years of guiding people through our home-delivered Reset Cleanse, we have learned a lot about what support people need, what works, and what doesn't. We developed the Juice Cleanse Reset Diet to provide a bridge for you to get from where you are now to where you want to be: the slimmer, younger-looking, more energetic, healthier you. Many of our celebrity clients have used our juices to prepare for a movie, slim down for a wedding, drop baby weight after the birth of their children, or get red-carpet ready. Professional athletes have enhanced their performance and rebuilt after injury, and many of our clients have used our Reset Cleanse products to reset their eating habits after letting them slide on vacation, to jump-start a weight-loss program, or to treat a health issue.

People have the most significant and lasting results when our three-day Reset Cleanse is used as part of a seven-day plan. We start with two days to prepare your body and mind for the cleanse, and then give you two days to ease back into eating solid food after the cleanse. We will tell you everything you need to know *before* you start cleansing, and we'll even give you a short quiz to help you determine what type of cleanse is right for you. (Don't worry, there are no wrong answers and our Juice Cleanse Reset Diet works for everyone, whether you've been eating junk food for the last twenty years or you eat completely raw, organic, and vegan.) And since we don't want to leave you hanging after you successfully complete the seven-day program, we give you lots of tips and advice for maintaining your new way of eating and living. And finally, since we all want to look our best before a special occasion (like a wedding, a high school reunion, or even a big work meeting), we've included three bonus resets that we call "supercharged resets"; these intensive three-day, ten-day, and twenty-one day programs will create dramatic results.

As you embark on this plan, you'll be amazed at how easy it is to follow, how satisfied you feel, and how much energy you have. You will also be surprised to experience an effortless change in your cravings and thoughts about food and what you put into your body. The Juice Cleanse Reset Diet is highly adaptable to any nutritional style. If you like chicken, you will continue to eat chicken. If you're a vegetarian, you won't need to introduce meat into your diet. You will simply learn how to eat in a way that keeps your body clean following your reset. You will also learn how to easily work exercise into your reset and how to sustain those eating and exercise habits for life.

This is a groundbreaking way to return your body to optimal health and fitness without depriving yourself of the nutrients you need or disrupting your daily routine. Our easy, accessible recipes and preparations are perfect for you anywhere, anytime. Seven days from now, when you reflect on how much better you look and feel, you'll realize that your results are sustainable for the rest of your life. Are you ready to reset? Let's get started!

one

WHY RESET?

> "The food you eat can either be the safest and most powerful form of medicine or the slowest form of poison."
>
> —Ann Wigmore, cofounder of Hippocrates Health Institute

We all have a different reason for starting a cleanse. What's yours?

Are you tired of waking up every morning with puffy eyes and swollen hands?

Have you been trying to lose that stubborn last ten pounds?

Do you frequently feel bloated and gassy?

Are you striving to look your best in the outfit you have chosen for an upcoming special occasion?

Would you love to regain the beautiful skin and hair of your youth?

Do you feel stressed, fatigued, and overwhelmed?

Do you binge eat and experience mood swings you can't control?

Do you want to look great in a bathing suit on a tropical vacation?

Are you ready to embark on a healthier lifestyle and eating plan?

Whatever your particular reason, your goal is to be your best self, and the Juice Cleanse Reset Diet is the bridge to your goal. We will give you a road map to achieve your ideal weight, rejuvenate your beauty, regain your health, or rev up your energy level. We will help you strip away and overcome all the obstacles in your way.

If you have tried other diets, eating plans, or protocols in the past with only limited success, or only to go back to your old bad habits, you're not alone. Keeping off the weight, and sticking to your resolution to eat healthier, is more than just a choice. Your body, habits, thought processes, and daily choices have been conditioned a certain way over days or months or years. Before you can change, you need to reset those patterns. No matter how hard you work at eating and exercising right, other programs can't get you what you want because they don't supply the *real* missing link.

The Juice Cleanse Reset Diet is a jump start to new habits and renewed health. "Resetting" your system is the single step that creates fewer cravings, lasting weight loss, increased energy, glowing skin, and a healthy body.

THE RESETS

While our bodies are generally very adept at removing toxins, sometimes all of the toxins in our food, the air we breathe, and the everyday products we use to clean our houses, wash our hair, and moisturize our skin are more than our bodies can handle. Different circumstances and toxins can overtax our digestive system and our cleansing organs. Maybe you have experienced the aftereffects of a night of too much drinking. It seems it takes the entire next day for your body to get rid of the toxins and for you to start feeling "normal" again. Or maybe you have been out to a great restaurant with friends and you overindulged in fried foods and dessert. That night, you have trouble sleeping because your stomach is rumbling and upset. Or you may have taken antibiotics and other drugs to help your body recover from an illness. As a result, your energy is low and you feel sluggish from residual chemicals.

These are occasional challenges to our bodies—drinking too much, overeating, taking medications—but imagine what happens when we constantly overload our bodies with various toxins. We constantly feel less than great. We become accustomed to feeling sluggish and having a tummy ache. Waking up with a headache or the sniffles seems completely normal. We get used to sleeping poorly and feeling tired. These toxins need to be cleaned out before we can stick to our resolve to be healthy. Each cell of your body—from your internal organs to your bones and muscles, skin and hair—needs enzymes, vitamins, and minerals to stay healthy and youthful. When those cells are filled with toxins, they have no room to take in enzymes, nutrients, and vitamins. Your cells cannot tap the full potential of those little powerhouses. Once the toxins have been flushed from your cells, however, your body will be receptive to all the nutritious goodness contained in the fruits and veggies in your juices or smoothies. And because the juicing and blending processes break up the cell walls of the produce, all of those nutrients are free to flood straight into your cells like liquid sunshine—rejuvenating, healing, nourishing, and resetting.

The Juice Cleanse Reset Diet helps your body rid itself of residual toxins and habits, and helps reset your attitude, taste buds, metabolism, cravings, digestive system, and weight. Toxin overload affects different people in different ways. It may affect your mental state, or it might manifest physically to the point of becoming detrimental to your health. Let's take a look at the seven resets. See which ones seem to fit your current situation most closely.

Reset Your Attitude and Your Mindset

When embarking on a new way of eating and fueling your body, it is important to reset your attitude. Your thought processes, habits, and mindset will have a huge impact on your chances of success. If you think you can succeed, your chances of success improve dramatically!

If you learn to love food and what it can do to help your body, you can stop those negative relationships with candy and desserts and junk food. Believe and embrace that the next seven days will change your life and reset your health.

Reset Your Energy

When you don't feed your body on a regular basis, or when you consume a lot of energy drinks or caffeine, or feed it processed, chemically engineered food, you actually sap your body of energy. Your body needs nutritious food to function properly and sustain you in your busy life. Over the next seven days, you will feed your body what it needs, avoid what it does not, and emerge energized.

Reset Your Metabolism

If you have not been eating four to six small meals a day, starting with a healthy nutrient-dense breakfast, your metabolism may be working against you. Once you train your body to expect nutrition every few hours, it will become accustomed to burning fuel rather than storing it. Your body will burn more calories and produce more energy.

Reset Your Taste Buds

When you consume a diet high in processed food, your taste buds get confused. They begin to prefer the taste of fried, battered, sugared food to natural food. Because foods that are processed or full of chemicals are generally void of nutrients, your body keeps craving more, because it isn't being nourished. No wonder diets in the past have been difficult! We will use the next seven days to reset your taste buds so that you will crave real, nutritious food.

Reset Your Digestive System

Too many people live with digestive issues and don't even know there is an easy cure. Our bodies do not know what to do with processed food. Your digestive system was not designed to filter out the excess hormones and antibiotics that may be contained in the meat, poultry, and dairy products you consume. You need fiber, a healthy digestive system, and real food for your body to operate properly. Once you rid yourself of the gunk, reset your system, and give your body what it needs, you will be amazed at how great you feel every day. You'll wish you had known it was this easy to feel good sooner.

Reset Your Weight

Throughout the diet, you will be pleased to notice that you're dropping excess pounds. As your body releases toxins, your abdomen will become leaner and less bloated. Your healthier cravings will help you continue to lose or maintain your perfect weight after the cleanse.

Reset Your Beauty

Radiant clear skin, full healthy hair, and bright rested eyes are all outer indications of beauty and reflections of inner health. When you look tired, your skin sags and is puffy and blemished, and your hair is limp or thinning, those are all indications that your body is suffering inside. Exposure to excess toxins, both from our food and from the environment, saps our beauty. On this diet, you will clean your body from the inside and learn to eat beauty-boosting food.

ANA M., MARKETING EXECUTIVE • I love drinking my green lemon juice from Ritual Wellness every morning and my spicy lemonade in the afternoons when I feel I need an energy boost. When I first began receiving weekly deliveries of juice each Monday morning, my husband didn't get it. He doesn't love vegetables and was put off by the color of the juice itself. We've been married for over ten years, so I know not to push him. He needs to discover some things for himself, in his own time.

Last month I went on a three-week trip to Italy with my mom. We had such a fun time together, seeing the sights, eating the delicious food and desserts, and drinking way too much fabulous wine from all of the vineyards we toured. Two days before we left Italy, I sent an email to Ritual Wellness asking if they could add the three-day Reset Cleanse to my normal delivery the following Monday. I knew that, although I had thoroughly enjoyed my indulgences, I wanted to get myself immediately back on track when I got home and drop the few pounds I could tell I had gained. And honestly, I was craving my green lemon juice! For the three weeks while I had been away, I had not stopped my weekly deliveries. I told my husband he could either freeze the juices for me to drink when I got home, or he could feel free to drink them himself.

When I got home, I was thrilled to find only a handful of juices in my freezer, and a husband requesting that I increase our weekly deliveries to include a green lemon juice for him each morning. I was even happier to drink nothing but juices for the next three days, get back to my normal routine, and fit back into my favorite jeans.

NEXT STEPS

As you embark on the Juice Cleanse Reset Diet, you will strip away old habits, thought patterns, and stored-up toxins to reset your body and your health. You do not need to stop your busy life or become a vegetarian or a vegan. You will just learn the best way to eat and live within your preferences. You will discover that not every calorie is created equal and that nutrient-dense foods can satisfy you like you never imagined.

You won't starve yourself or even feel hungry. In the first few days, you will eat delicious foods frequently, and drink yummy smoothies and juices that you will learn to make for yourself. By changing your diet to include whole foods that contain natural fiber, beneficial fat, and protein, you will notice that you need less food to feel satisfied and you will stay satisfied longer. This isn't a crash diet. This is a reset.

In the next chapter, we'll tell you everything you need to know to get ready to cleanse. If you're anxious to get started and just want to jump in with both feet, you can skip ahead to the test on page 42 to find out what sort of cleanse you need and then head to chapter 3 to start the precleanse phase. However, the information that follows helps you prepare your life, your kitchen, and your mindset for cleansing, and gives you the start you need to be successful. Let's go!

two

GETTING READY TO CLEANSE

"Begin with the end in mind."

—Stephen R. Covey, author of *The 7 Habits of Highly Effective People*

Imagine that you work in a messy and disorganized office. Stacks of old paperwork, new projects, bills, folders, books, and magazines cover every surface. The desk drawers are equally stuffed and the filing cabinets are overflowing. When you walk in, it feels cluttered and overwhelming, you waste a lot of time each day just looking for the right files, and you get easily distracted by all the junk.

Then one day, you make the decision to get organized. There will be no more piles! You will touch each piece of paper only once. You will open the mail, read it, and either toss it in the trash or place it in an appropriate file. You will pay your bills immediately, and then file the payment stub. You'll line up all of your books in a bookshelf on one wall, and you'll either read your magazines right away and then place them in a storage folder or recycle them. You will frame your photos and hang them neatly along the walls.

Sounds great, right? But to do this, you first need to sort through all those piles, empty those drawers, and cull through the file cabinets. The desk and bookshelves need to be cleared of clutter to make way for the organized items. The process will take some time and attention, and everything will seem even more cluttered at first. You may be tempted to shove everything back in the drawers when you find out a colleague is coming over for a meeting!

But if you resist the urge to give up and really go through the cleansing process, you will have a much better chance of keeping your office organized going forward. And you will feel so much better. The energy you previously used to hunt down a particular letter or document can now be spent on getting your work done more efficiently so you can do more pleasurable activities outside of the office. The frustration you felt at being disorganized will disappear. You will be so inspired by your new clean office that it will be easier to keep it clean. The systems you put in place to organize your work will allow you to keep your office organized. Sure, every now and then, you might let a stack of mail sit for a day or two, but because you have a method for sorting and dispatching your mail quickly, you're able to get right back on top of it, keeping it neat and organized.

Your body is a little bit like that imaginary office. Once you let your good habits slide and things get messy, it seems easier and less painful to keep the status quo. You promise yourself to eat cleaner and exercise more, but without a foundation in place to keep you organized and accountable, you slip back into your old habits. In this chapter, we'll tell you how to build a structure (like having a process for sorting the mail and filing your paperwork) so you can keep your body clean, healthy, and functioning efficiently during and after your cleanse.

PREPPING FOR YOUR CLEANSE

Have you ever done a cleanse before? How did it make you feel? Were you able to complete it? If not, what were the reasons you failed? Perhaps your cravings got the best of you, or you felt light-headed and tired, or perhaps you found yourself hungry. Maybe your resolve wasn't that strong, or you didn't see results fast enough on the scale, so you threw in the towel.

This chapter will teach you how to prepare for your cleanse, make it easier, and ensure your success. There are three phases to the Juice Cleanse Reset Diet—the precleanse phase, the juice-cleanse phase, and the postcleanse phase—and all are equally important. Throughout the three phases, you will be resetting your body for the rest of your life.

Benefits of the Juice Cleanse Reset Diet

Reset Your Attitude and Your Mindset: You will have a better attitude toward food and nutrition, and be able to fight off urges and cravings. You will have a strong desire to continue on this path to a healthier you for the rest of your life.

Reset Your Energy: You will be surprised at how your energy levels soar and that afternoon slump disappears.

Reset Your Metabolism: You will have a faster, more efficient metabolism, which will help you burn more calories and shed excess weight.

Reset Your Taste Buds: You will crave more of what Mother Nature has to offer and crave less processed food.

Reset Your Digestive System: Your body will be more efficient at using and absorbing nutrients, vitamins, and enzymes and will be quicker at eliminating waste.

Reset Your Weight: You will lose a few pounds, and will continue to lose more as you move forward.

Reset Your Beauty: You will be thrilled with your glowing skin, clearer eyes, and rejuvenated beauty.

Successfully achieving your desired resets requires you to prepare for the Juice Cleanse Reset Diet. The following section gives you all of the information you need in order to plan for success both during the program and for the long haul. It's true that following the Juice Cleanse Reset Diet will take a commitment of your time and energy. But it's also true that the results will be worth every ounce of energy that you expend! We not only review planning for success on the program, but also give you a plan to clean out your cupboards as well as the information you need to navigate through the supermarket with ease and confidence.

Plan for Success

The easiest way to dramatically change your diet is to completely plan out your meals ahead of time and get all the grocery shopping done *before* you start. If you have a busy schedule, grabbing food on the go is one of the most challenging habits to break. It's also a change that makes a huge impact on your long-term success.

Get cozy with your calendar and pick a chunk of time that you can dedicate to shopping and prepping your food for the week. If you can carve out this time to plan your meals, you will be amazed at how easy the issue of food becomes for the rest of your week. This approach to shopping and prepping not only works well for the Juice Cleanse Reset Diet, but it's also an effective way to handle mealtime after the reset, while you maintain your new way of eating.

Clean Out Your Cupboards

It's time to clear your kitchen of all processed items that disguise themselves as food and to stock your pantry with only the essentials needed for your seven-day reset. Staying on track will be much easier if you get rid of any foods that could be detrimental to your success. If you hesitate to ditch the salty chips, sweet candy, or that peanut jar that you visit too many times per day, those items likely pose the

Meal-Planning Tips

- Plan your meals in advance. Select from the recipes in this book or subscribe to our blog at www.ritualwellness.com for more recipe ideas. If you don't enjoy cooking, choose two recipes to make each week and make double so you have four meals ready to go.

- Make a few dishes that can be eaten several ways. For example, the roasted veggies you make for dinner on Sunday can be added to a lunch salad on Monday. And leftovers from the rotisserie chicken you bought for Tuesday night can be used in all sorts of dishes, including the Chicken Salad (page 190), Butter Lettuce Tacos (page 195), or Roasted Veggie and Chicken Salad (page 186) recipes found in this book.

- If a recipe calls for you to prepare a sauce, make a big batch and freeze what you don't use in ice cube trays. Next time you make the recipe, defrost enough for that meal. This is a big time-saver!

- Make a big batch of steel-cut oatmeal in the slow cooker on Sunday night and have it for the week.

- Stock up on organic frozen fruit and frozen spinach or kale for easy smoothies.

greatest threat of derailing your success. Do not keep any of these foods in the house during your reset! It's time to reclaim control and overcome the power that these foods have over you!

If you take the time to acknowledge the challenge this food causes for you, recognize your conscious choice to say no to this food, celebrate your decision, and reflect on how empowered you feel, you can release the control that this food has over you. The next time this food is in your path (keeping it out of your home doesn't mean you'll never see it again), your odds of passing on it are much better. Perhaps more importantly, if you do choose to indulge in it, you'll be making a conscious choice to do so rather than reverting back to an old habit.

How to Overcome Temptation

- Acknowledge the challenge this food causes for you.

- Recognize that you can make a conscious choice to say no to this food.

- Pause and celebrate your decision to prioritize your health.

- Reflect on how empowering the decision to say no to temptation is and sit with the feeling.

Buy and Eat Real Food

The greatest thing that you can do as you begin this cleanse is to dedicate yourself to the idea of eating real food. Yep, you read that correctly: "Eat. Real. Food." Michael Pollan coined this phrase and it has been restated a hundred different ways, but the sentiment is the same.

Many modern-day health issues are caused or exacerbated by the shift in eating habits that has taken us further and further away from food as it is in its most natural state. Choosing to eat real food ensures that you take in the nutrients your body needs in order to operate properly. Chemicals and additives, which are foreign to your body and cannot be utilized, cause weight gain, health challenges, energy depletion, and allergy issues.

AMY J., WORKING MOTHER OF THREE • I'm a fully recovered sugar addict! Thanks to the Juice Cleanse Reset Diet and following Lori and Marra's guidance to say good-bye to my trigger foods, I finally feel back in charge of what I feed my body. For years, I struggled with massive sugar cravings, mood swings (my poor husband), and generally feeling out of control when it came to food. I committed to the reset program, and I can honestly say that it's the best decision I ever made for my health. The sugar withdrawal was intense during the first few days, so intense that I am certain I would have caved in if I still had a stash of sweets in the cupboards. Thank goodness I didn't because today, nine months post-reset, I still feel amazing and I am back to my prepregnancy weight. Best of all, if I choose to have a bite of dessert, I can stop there instead of slipping into the sugar-eating tailspin that used to happen after what started out as "just a bite."

Today, nearly everything with a label screams something at you: "Low-carb!" "High-protein!" "Vitamin-fortified!" "All-natural!" "Trans fat free!" or "Fat-free!" There was a time when no one, other than food scientists, thought of food as the macronutrients that made it up. Before refined flour started to replace whole grains, bread was bread, period. Still, it wasn't until the 1980s that we began thinking of bread as a carbohydrate instead of an essential part of a sandwich. This shift toward viewing food as the nutrients rather than food has greatly contributed to the huge mess currently lining supermarket shelves.

Over the years, bread has become even more complicated. (We'll stick with our example of bread even though there are endless examples of pure and simple foods that now come filled with chemicals, preservatives, and additives.) Today you can buy bread that is low carb, high protein, fortified with various vitamins, or even grain free! The result? Many people are overwhelmed by the decision to buy something as simple as bread.

Bread: Then and Now

Here's the ingredient list of a basic loaf of bread when your great-grandparents ate it:

flour • yeast • water • salt

Here's the ingredient list of one of today's most popular store-bought breads:

flour • yeast • sugar • wheat gluten • wheat bran • soybean oil • honey • molasses • salt • vinegar • calcium carbonate • calcium propionate • sodium stearoyl lactylate • calcium sulfate • mono calcium phosphate • yeast extract • soy lecithin • azodicarbonamide • calcium dioxide • soy flour • whey

Store-bought bread is one of the many examples of a once-simple food that has been manipulated into something that barely resembles food any longer. Everywhere you look, processed, chemically altered, and engineered nutrition is trickily disguised as food.

The good news is that by following the Juice Cleanse Reset Diet, you will reset your palate and be better able to identify the difference between real food and artificially engineered products. During the days after your Reset Cleanse, a strawberry will taste sweet and delicious, as nature intended. A store-bought, prepackaged cookie filled with refined sweeteners and shelf life–extending additives will taste unnatural and processed—because it is!

Buy Organic

During the cleanse, it's imperative that you use as close to 100 percent organic ingredients as possible. Conventional foods come with a heavy burden of pesticides, or hormones and antibiotics in the case of animal products, none of which is conducive to cleansing. While our dream scenario is for you to consume organic foods all of the time, we're more flexible on this after your cleanse phase is complete. It's nearly impossible to dine out or engage in social situations and stick to a fully organic diet. Eating 100 percent organic is a greater challenge than eating 100 percent vegan! With this in mind, the time to make organic food a priority is when you're eating at home.

There are certain fruits and vegetables that you should always consume in their organic form. The Environmental Working Group (EWR) puts together a list every year called the "Dirty Dozen." The Dirty Dozen is your guide to the most toxic conventional fruits and vegetables. The potential toxic load, as reported by the EWR, is huge,

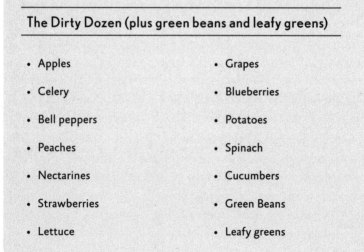

The Dirty Dozen (plus green beans and leafy greens)

- Apples
- Celery
- Bell peppers
- Peaches
- Nectarines
- Strawberries
- Lettuce

- Grapes
- Blueberries
- Potatoes
- Spinach
- Cucumbers
- Green Beans
- Leafy greens

with residues from up to sixty-four different pesticides containing carcinogens, neurotoxins, hormone disruptors, developmental or reproductive toxins, and toxins that are killing honey bees.

The EWR added two more items to the 2012 list but didn't want to abandon the catchy phrase of "dirty dozen." Instead, they created an addendum: "plus green beans and leafy greens" (think kale and collard greens). EWR warns that these new additions "contain pesticide residue of special concern" because they are commonly contaminated with insecticides that "are toxic to the nervous system."

EWR also warns against eating conventional corn in the United States because corn is one of the most genetically engineered crops and is not required to be labeled as such. Long story short—in addition to the famous Dirty Dozen, stay away from toxic greens and genetically engineered corn by choosing organic!

Why Washing Is Not Enough

Many people have been falsely led to believe that washing produce well brings conventionally grown produce up to par with organically grown produce. We have even heard juice bars claim that their products are pesticide free because they are washed thoroughly, despite using conventional produce. Unfortunately, this is not the case! Since fruits and vegetables have pores, pesticides can infiltrate produce on a cellular level and cannot be fully removed through washing. According to the National Pesticide Information Center, "no washing method is 100 percent effective for removing all pesticide residues."

To spot organic food, look for:

- USDA Organic: Trust it. Buy it. Ninety-five percent or more of the ingredients must have been grown or processed without synthetic fertilizers or pesticides (among other standards). In the case of meat and dairy, this seal also indicates the products are growth-hormone and antibiotic free!

- Made with Organic Ingredients: This statement in conjunction with the USDA seal means the product must contain a minimum of 70 percent organic ingredients. The label will indicate which ingredients are organic and tell you the percentage of organic ingredients used.

Be cautious of:

- Organic (without certification): Some organic companies choose not to get certified due to a lack of resources. If it's labeled organic but not certified, you must decide whether or not you trust the source. In instances when a product claims to be organic with no seal, base your purchasing decision on your own research.

- Conventional: If a product says nothing one way or the other on the subject of organic, it is conventional, meaning it is *not* organic in any way.

- All Natural: The FDA has not developed a definition for the term *natural*. Unless otherwise stated, consider something that claims to be "natural" to be in the same arena as conventional. Even items with high-fructose corn syrup (HFCS) as the first ingredient can claim "all natural" on the label because the HFCS is a derivative of corn.

- Organic When Possible: You may see this in a retail establishment/restaurant. Organic is nearly always possible, but it's almost always more expensive. Ask the shop or restaurant owner what their standards are for determining "when possible" because the truth is that it's nearly always possible, at a price.

- Local: Local has no relevance to the term *organic*. A pesticide is a pesticide, even if it comes from your own backyard.

- Wild-crafted: This is a new buzzword in the food and supplement arena. Wild-crafted is the practice of harvesting plants from their natural or "wild" habitat, for food or medicinal purposes. However, the term *wild-crafted* has no real significance as to whether it is organic or not. Food suppliers are stretching the term to mean picked from the plant while leaving the plant intact, even if the "habitat" is a pesticide-ridden farm.

And when it comes to produce:

- Fruits and vegetables: Fruits and vegetables are naked—the best way to eat your food. This means no packaging. It also means no place for that beautiful USDA organic seal. For your fruits and veggies, learn the following number codes, which usually appear on a sticker.

  Five-digit PLU (price look-up) starting with 9: Organic. Yes, buy it.

  Five-digit PLU starting with 8: Genetically modified (see page 37). Do not buy it.

  Four-digit PLU: Conventionally grown with the use of pesticides. If there is not a frozen, organic variety available, conventional produce is still better than processed foods.

Vote with Your Dollars

Remember that you truly do vote with your dollars. Every time you choose organic over the conventional alternative, your voice is heard loud and clear by the supermarkets, food distributors, and farmers. You hold the power to make a difference in our food system.

If you're committed to doing your reset, it's important for you to use organic produce. You're putting forth a huge effort to do something good for your health and if you choose conventional, you may be unleashing a toxic burden on your cells through the form of concentrated pesticides in the fruits and veggies.

While calorie for calorie conventional and organic may be the same, in addition to the benefit of avoiding toxic pesticides, organic produce has been reported to deliver more antioxidants than its conventional counterparts. A 2011 article by Gene E. Lester and Robert A. Saftner, published in the *Journal of Agricultural and Food Chemistry*, references two separate studies that demonstrated organic vegetables to have between 15 to 25 percent higher levels of some antioxidants than their conventional counterparts.

Think of antioxidants as nature's equivalent to the human immune system. You probably know that taking antibiotics repeatedly weakens your own defenses in the form of antioxidants. Rather than increasing your immune system by building antibodies, your body gets used to relying on external antibiotics. In a similar way, when crops are continuously flooded with pesticides to keep bugs away, the plants have no reason to build up their own defenses. These defenses are beneficial to humans, and when the plants lack defense-related compounds, the produce is less nutritious. Choosing organic helps you limit your toxic load and increases your nutrient consumption.

If organic produce is unavailable or is outside of your budget, we highly recommend buying frozen organic produce. This is a great option and is definitely our recommendation over conventional produce.

Choose Healthy Dairy, Meats, and Seafood

Because we're natural health enthusiasts with an affinity for green juices, people expect us to promote a vegan lifestyle. We don't. Even crazier, we believe it's okay to eat meat, even red meat. Mind blowing, we know. Before you get too excited and go on a burger-eating escapade, let us explain a bit further. While we don't think that being an omnivore automatically means you're doomed to obesity and disease, we do think that you should consume animal products responsibly and sparingly.

With this in mind, your consumption of animal protein should be limited to 10 to 15 percent of your diet. This quantity allows you to reap the nutritional benefits of animal protein, like amino acids and B vitamins, without derailing your diet plan.

We strongly urge you to choose organic meat, poultry, and dairy. It can be challenging to find restaurants that serve organic options. Rather than vowing to never eat out again, a great solution is to order a vegetarian option or to select wild-caught fish. The pesticides on your veggies or salads are not ideal either, but they are the better option when compared to hormone- and antibiotic-filled meat and dairy.

When eating at home, you have more control over what you eat and how it's prepared. In choosing meat for at-home meals, select organic and cook at low temperatures. Cooking at low temperatures protects you against cancer-causing heterocyclic amines (HCAs) and polycyclic aromatic hydrocarbons (PAHs). These chemicals form when muscle meat, including beef, pork, fish, and poultry, are cooked using high-temperature methods, such as pan frying or grilling directly over an open flame. If you like your meat charred, we urge you to consider the health detriments of these toxins and try some of the slow-cooking recipes in this book.

Hormone free, grass fed, natural—the list is long and the messages on labels can easily cause confusion. Choosing the healthiest options requires you to be able to decipher the many different labels and key phrases commonly found on dairy, beef, poultry, and eggs.

To help you make smart decisions, we have broken down many of the terms used on these products. Understanding the differences among these labels will help you navigate your way through the supermarket aisle with confidence.

Look for:

- USDA Organic (dairy, eggs, meat, poultry): Cattle have never been treated with antibiotics. Feed is organic and GMO free. Chickens are only given antibiotics in the case of infection. In contrast, conventionally raised chicks are administered antibiotics on a routine basis.

- AGA-Certified Grass Fed (beef, dairy, lamb): Takes the USDA standards to a higher level. Means the animal was born and raised in the United States, fed 100 percent grass, and was never given antibiotics or hormones. A comprehensive review of over three decades of research was written in 2010 by California State University, Chico, and was published in *Nutrition Journal*, verifying that grass-fed beef has lower levels of cholesterol and unhealthy fats, as well as higher levels of vitamins A and E and omega-3 fatty acids.

- 100% Grass Fed, USDA Process Verified (beef, dairy, lamb): Animals were fed 100 percent grass and forage. Does not exclude use of antibiotics.

- Animal Welfare Approved (dairy, eggs, meat, poultry): The highest animal welfare standards of any third-party auditing program. Antibiotics are allowed to treat sick animals only. Slaughter and milking are only allowed after antibiotics are out of the animal's system.

- Wild Caught (fish): Farmed fish are typically fed antibiotics. Wild-caught fish are not. There is no such thing as organic fish. If you see a claim for organic fish, it's bogus.

Avoid Hormones and Antibiotics in Your Food

Although the FDA regulates the amount of antibiotics and hormones contained in conventional dairy products, we wonder: should any amount be allowed? Recombinant bovine growth hormone (rBGH) is a genetically engineered form of the natural growth hormone produced by cows. Injecting cows with this artificial hormone expedites their growth rate and boosts their milk production by 10 percent, but it also greatly increases their incidence of mastitis. Mastitis is an infection that must be treated with antibiotics. You can see how this practice can quickly become a self-perpetuating cycle of injecting hormones and antibiotics.

Products labeled as rBGH free are often labeled as antibiotic free as well, since antibiotics are less likely to be needed when the cows are not injected with hormones. Due to the clear association between rBGH and human antibiotic resistance, as well as an increased risk of breast cancer, colon cancer, and prostate cancer in humans, the additive has been banned in Canada, Japan, New Zealand, Australia, and the European Union. Yet, we are still using rBGH in the United States. We recommend you stay away from this hormone completely.

Be cautious of:

- Natural: Term is not regulated and has little meaning. In reference to meat, "natural" can be claimed if there is no food coloring. GMO feed, antibiotics, and hormones are allowed.

- Antibiotic Free/No Antibiotic Residues: Since the USDA does not regulate this term, it does not hold much meaning.

- rBGH Free (dairy): Indicates that the cows have not been treated with recombinant bovine growth hormone. rBGH is used in conventional cattle raising to massively increase milk production by the cow. Mastitis (inflammation of the udders, often caused by infection) has been linked to rBGH treatment. Conventional cows given rBGH are pumped full of antibiotics. This seal does not say anything about placing limitations on the use of antibiotics, but there may be a smaller need for antibiotics in rBGH-free cows.

- Free Range, Free Roaming, or Cage Free (poultry, eggs): Typically, the chickens are uncaged inside barns or warehouses and have some degree of outdoor access, but there are no requirements for the amount, duration, or quality of outdoor access. No restrictions regarding what the birds can be fed or regarding the use of antibiotics and hormones. Look for free range in combination with the USDA seal for your best option.

Many health food markets sell free-range, USDA organic, 100 percent grass-fed beef. Today websites like www.eatwild.com allow you to search for responsible dairy and cattle farms in your area, providing a great option to purchase meat and dairy products that satisfy all of your requirements without breaking the bank. Many of the small farms that offer online purchasing and home delivery give discounts if you buy in bulk. Consider getting together with a few friends or neighbors to invest in the best quality at the best price.

Seafood is no exception to the rule that knowledge is the first tenet of a healthy eating plan. You must be an educated consumer in order to select your seafood. While seafood can be very healthy, it also can be contaminated with mercury and other toxins. Additionally, overfishing of certain types of fish has a detrimental environmental impact. Still, there are many very healthy seafood options that are perfectly safe and beneficial to include in your diet.

Seafood Watch is a great resource where you can find out about safe, healthy, and sustainable seafood options. Visit the website www.montereybayaquarium.org/cr/seafoodwatch.aspx and view their seafood recommendations. For your convenience, they offer a pocket guide and a downloadable application.

Avoid (due to high toxin levels):

- Most U.S. and Canadian farmed fish of all types. Farmed shellfish is the exception and is often safe to eat.

Limit (due to high mercury levels):

- Swordfish
- Tuna (fresh and canned)
- Marlin
- Orange roughy

Enjoy:

- Wild salmon
- Striped bass
- Alaskan halibut
- Anchovies
- Crab

Stay Away from Genetically Modified Foods

Do you eat conventional meal replacement bars or cereal, fast food, or any nonorganic processed foods? If so, chances are high that you consume genetically modified organisms (GMOs). The World Health Organization defines GMOs as "organisms in which the genetic material (DNA) has been altered in a way that does not occur naturally."

According to the Institute for Responsible Technology, there are many reasons to be concerned about genetically engineered foods, including a lack of proof about their long-term effects on humans, their potential to disrupt natural growing cycles, and the allergen risks. GMOs represent one more way that big companies create foods that are further away from their natural forms.

A Word on Raw

If you're a dairy eater, seek out raw milk and cheese in your local markets. Most milk is heat pasteurized, which reduces the nutritional quality and decreases your body's ability to digest it well. Studies done by the Department of Food Hygiene and Technology in Córdoba, Spain, are among many that have shown that milk has a decrease in manganese, copper, and iron after heat treatment. The FDA has acknowledged that pasteurization destroys a substantial portion of the vitamin C in milk, and sterilization is also known to significantly impair the bioactivity of vitamin B_6 contained in milk. Heating juice damages the enzymes in it, making it harder for your body to absorb the nutrients. The same goes for milk. The heating of milk during pasteurization damages its inherent lactase (the naturally occurring enzyme needed to break down lactose). Consuming lactose without the presence of lactase causes digestive grief for many people. The Weston A. Price Foundation conducted an informal survey of more than seven hundred families and determined that more than 80 percent of those diagnosed with lactose intolerance no longer suffer from symptoms after switching to raw milk.

It is illegal to sell raw milk in many states. In states where the sale of raw milk is prohibited, you may be able to purchase raw milk directly from a local farm through a cow share program. Participating in a cow share program typically requires an upfront payment of around $75. This payment covers the costs for the farmer to board, feed, care for, and milk the cow. In exchange, you receive weekly deliveries of raw milk. You can find a list of participating farms online at www.eatwild.com.

While it is evident that raw milk offers substantial nutritional benefits, it is important to realize that raw milk has not been treated to kill potential pathogens. For your safety, if you are pregnant, nursing, or have a weakened immune system, you should consult your doctor before consuming raw dairy products.

A shocking 70 percent of processed foods sold in the United States today contain genetically modified organisms. Breakfast cereals; meal replacement, protein, or snack bars; and salad dressings are all commonly consumed foods that frequently contain GMOs. Conventional (nonorganic) corn, sugar, soy protein, cornstarch, and vegetable oil used in U.S. products almost always come from genetically modified crops.

Foods containing GMOs first hit supermarket shelves in the early 1990s. Due to lack of testing and long-term study of human health and environmental effects, sixty-one countries currently mandate the labeling of GMOs and dozens more have banned the import, sale, use, and planting of GMOs. Unfortunately, the United States currently has no regulations around the labeling of GMOs in food. Recently, a large consumer movement has demanded labeling GM foods within the United States. Thankfully, responsible businesses and consumer advocates are working to get GMOs in foods labeled. Whole Foods is leading the charge toward total food transparency in the United States, requiring that all GM foods in their stores be labeled by 2018.

- Until the FDA mandates labeling of GMOs, look for the Non-GMO Project seal. Learn more at www.nongmoproject.org.

Limit Your Consumption of Soy

Although soy food sales increased from $1 billion to more than $5.2 billion between 1996 and 2011, soy has now fallen from grace. A few short years ago, we were told to consume soy to prevent cancer, heart disease, and osteoporosis, and to fight inflammation. However, today research points to soy as a cause of estrogen-sensitive cancers, thyroid disease, and mineral deficiency.

What happened? Let's start with the thought that not all soy is created equally. As the demand for soy increased and big food companies began using it in all sorts of products, it became a highly processed crop. A staggering 90 percent of soy in the United States has been genetically modified! Just as corn is widely used in the food industry because it yields the most inexpensive form of carbohydrate, soy is abused in the modern food industry because it provides the most inexpensive form of fat and protein.

When it comes to consuming soy:

- Avoid overconsumption of hidden soy by removing processed food from your diet.

- Choose USDA organic to avoid genetically altered soy.

- Eat soy in moderation.

- Edamame and soybeans are the least processed forms of soy and are highly beneficial.

- Fermented soy products, like miso and tempeh, are great choices because the fermentation process neutralizes phytic acids, which may interfere with the absorption of minerals.

- Tofu and soy milk are good options as well, but they typically undergo more processing than edamame and tempeh do.

Let Quality Be Your Guide

Registered dietician Ashley Koff, who has given her stamp of approval to our home-delivered Reset Cleanse, coined the term *qualitarian* and we think it's brilliant. According to Ashley, *qualitarian* means, first and foremost, "that you choose to be the gatekeeper for what goes into your body. That you don't feel deprived but rather empowered when you turn down a veggie burger with genetically engineered ingredients or hexane and enjoy one made from organic quinoa and mushrooms or a wild salmon burger or a grass-fed burger. It also means saying no to a ready-to-eat salad of chemically sprayed lettuces in favor of cooking your own organic broccoli. And it means taking pride in being smarter than the front of a package or a commercial." The foundation of all sound eating philosophies is built on eating high-quality pure food.

Whether you're a vegan, vegetarian, pescetarian, or omnivore has little to do with whether you're eating a low-nutrient, high-crap diet. As a vegan, you could include lots of genetically engineered corn and soy products. As a vegetarian, you could overdose on the rBST in the creamer you dump in your morning coffee, in your grilled cheese at lunch, and again on your post-dinner pint of ice cream. As a pescetarian, you could fill your plate with toxin-ridden, farm-raised fish and pesticide-filled veggies. As an omnivore, you could eat hormone- and antibiotic-laden poultry or beef. The point is that none of these terms automatically equates with healthy. Whichever category you fit into, achieving your optimum health requires you to fill your diet with the highest quality foods that fit into your chosen lifestyle.

WHAT'S YOUR TYPE?

For centuries, people have used fasting—whether for spiritual reasons or to clear addictions, heal ailments, improve mental clarity, or increase energy—as a way to give the body a break and to embrace the new. Historically, fasting involves consuming only water, so the energy typically used for digestion can be saved. However, a water fast—which provides zero nutrients—doesn't generally work with the demanding, fast-paced lifestyle most of us lead. So we have developed a way for you get all of the benefits of fasting (and more), while also nourishing your body with whole foods!

Although the Juice Cleanse Reset Diet begins with a seven-day plan (or perhaps longer, depending on how long you stay in each phase), we teach you the skills to reset for life. We want you to pay attention to how you feel each day throughout the program in order to better understand your own body, thoughts, cravings, taste, and attitude. The key to making positive changes begins with understanding where your health is now.

Depending on your current lifestyle and habits, you may have one obstacle, or you may have many. For some of you, the issue is that you don't really know what to eat, because there is so much conflicting information from various experts. For others, you have just gotten into bad habits. For still others, you may make healthy choices most of the time, but occasionally you lapse (for example, you just got back from a vacation where you indulged a little too much). Depending on where you are currently, you may have only a minimal amount of toxins in your body, or you may be storing them in all of your cells.

The short test that follows will help you determine your "type," which, in turn, will indicate how you should approach your individual cleanse program for maximum results. Your current habits and lifestyle will impact whether you need to reset your attitude and mindset, your energy level, your metabolism, your taste buds, your digestive system, your weight, your beauty, or all seven.

THE TEST

Choose the answers below that best match your lifestyle. Choose only one answer for each question.

How do you feel about your current weight?
   A: I am at or within five pounds of my ideal weight.
   B: I can't seem to lose that last ten pounds!
   C: I seem to struggle and yo-yo with a twenty-pound swing.
   D: I am thirty or more pounds overweight.

How often do you eat fruits and veggies?
   A: Nearly every meal includes fruit or vegetables.
   B: I eat some type of fruit or vegetable pretty much every day
   C: I rarely eat fruit or vegetables.
   D: I just don't like vegetables.

Do you exercise?
- **A:** I work out three to five times per week.
- **B:** I fit in workouts intermittently, when my schedule allows, at least once or twice per week.
- **C:** I don't work out, but my job and life keep me pretty active.
- **D:** I lead a very sedentary lifestyle.

How many times do you drink alcohol per week?
- **A:** I don't drink any alcohol.
- **B:** Only on special occasions.
- **C:** I try to limit my drinking to the weekends rather than during the week.
- **D:** I have a couple of drinks with dinner most every evening.

What do think when you see the word *natural* on a label?
- **A:** I ignore it and look for the USDA symbol.
- **B:** *Natural* means no dyes or chemicals, right?
- **C:** Isn't *natural* the same as organic?
- **D:** I've never thought about it before.

How often do you drink water?
- **A:** I'm never without it.
- **B:** I have a couple of glasses a day.
- **C:** Once in a while, but I prefer other drinks.
- **D:** Almost never, only when I don't have other choices.

How often do you eat sweets like cookies, candy, or pastries?
- **A:** I never eat sugar.
- **B:** On special occasions.
- **C:** Once or twice a week.
- **D:** At least once a day.

How many cups of coffee do you drink per day?

A: I never drink coffee.

B: Two or three times a week.

C: I have one cup of coffee every morning.

D: Several throughout the day.

How often do you eat fried food?

A: Almost never.

B: Only occasionally, when I eat out at a restaurant.

C: A few times a week.

D: Most every day, since most of my meals are on the go.

How often do you consume sodas (including diet) and energy drinks?

A: Never.

B: Once in a while, as a treat.

C: One every day.

D: More than two every day.

How many servings of red meat do you eat per week?

A: I never eat it.

B: I only eat red meat on occasion.

C: A couple of times per week.

D: Most days.

How often do you consume dairy products like milk, cheese, and yogurt?

A: I try to avoid them.

B: A few times per week.

C: Daily.

D: A few times a day.

Do you take any probiotic or digestive supplements?
    A: I take a supplement every day.
    B: I eat yogurt every day.
    C: I eat yogurt several times a week.
    D: I am not sure I know what they are.

Do you drink juice?
    A: Yes, I make my own fruit and vegetable blends every day.
    B: I go to the juice bar a couple of times a week.
    C: There is always a carton of juice from the supermarket in my fridge.
    D: I rarely drink any type of juice.

When eating out, which dressing would you choose on your salad?
    A: Olive oil and lemon or vinegar.
    B: Vinaigrette on the side.
    C: Whatever dressing it comes with.
    D: Ranch, blue cheese, or anything creamy.

To score, add up the number of A, B, C, and D answers. If you have:

    Mostly As, you are type 1

    Mostly Bs, you are type 2

    Mostly Cs, you are type 3

    Mostly Ds, you are type 4

Type 1: You are the health enthusiast who has gotten off track and needs to reset to your normal healthy eating. For you, the Juice Cleanse Reset Diet will be more about resetting your taste buds and your attitude. You may have gotten accustomed to the taste of processed food, and you may be making bad choices unconsciously. You should follow the Juice Cleanse Reset Diet as presented here and spend two days in the precleanse phase. After the cleanse, you will find yourself naturally craving healthier foods and find it easier to make better choices.

Type 2: You are the weekend warrior who tends to eat well during the week and indulge on the weekend, but needs a reset to make more consistently healthy choices. You will need to spend three days in the precleanse phase to clear your body of the remnants of too much caffeine, alcohol, or processed food. You probably won't need to worry about detox symptoms, but by precleansing for this amount of time, you will reset your attitude, taste buds, metabolism, and digestive system to make your cleanse as enjoyable, easy, and effective as possible.

Type 3: You are the average person eating the standard American diet (SAD), which is a diet high in processed food and animal fats, and low in fiber, complex carbohydrates, and plant-based foods. Depending on some of your habits involving caffeine, sugar, and processed food, you should spend four days in the precleanse phase. You will want to reset your attitude, energy level, taste buds, and digestive system, and perhaps your weight and beauty as well. You have probably been eating too much processed food and not enough real, live food. You may be accustomed to eating only small amounts of food all day and then a huge dinner at night. In the precleanse phase, we will get your metabolism going in the morning, keep it on track all day long, and wean you off caffeine and sugar before you begin the juice cleanse, to help you avoid unpleasant detox symptoms like nausea and headaches.

Type 4: You are the junk food junkie who needs to completely overhaul your diet and reset for a healthier life. You will find that you may need to reset your attitude, energy level, metabolism, taste buds, digestive system, beauty, and weight. Your current eating habits may have you feeling sluggish and overweight, and you may not even like the taste of healthy food. We recommend that you spend seven days in the precleanse phase. If you try to rush the process, you may experience headaches, nausea, and irritability, and may not even want to continue with your juices. During the precleanse phase, we will begin the detox process in a mild way, and will start resetting your attitude and taste buds to prepare you for the juices.

The point of the quiz was not to make you feel good or bad about your current eating habits. We want to help you find your starting place. Each person's definition of a healthy eater is different (whether you are—or are not—one), so we want to help you easily define yourself for the purposes of the Juice Cleanse Reset Diet. Now that you've discovered your type, you're ready to begin the precleanse phase. Let's get going!

three

THE PRECLEANSE PHASE

"Don't let what you cannot do interfere with what you can do."

—Coach John Wooden

Depending on your daily choices and lifestyle, you may be storing a lot of toxins that will come up, and out, during the Juice Cleanse Reset Diet. And that might get messy. If you go straight from a diet of manufactured, chemically treated fast food to nutritious, real liquid food, all sorts of unpleasant things may happen. You may get a headache from the lack of caffeine, or a rash or nausea from all those chemicals coming to the surface at once. You may also be grumpy or tired or irritable as your hormones struggle to regulate themselves.

To avoid the nasty possibility of dealing with all of these toxin-related issues at once, we will walk you through a three-step process in this program. First, you'll ease off the junk through the precleanse phase (discussed below), where, depending on what type you are, you will stay for two to seven days. Then, when your body is ready, you'll start your juice-cleanse phase (see chapter 4), where you'll stay for three or more days, depending on whether you're making juice or smoothies. Finally, you'll finish with a postcleanse phase (see chapter 5), through which you'll reintroduce healthy foods to solidify your new habits.

The precleanse is the first formal phase of the Juice Cleanse Reset Diet and is very important. In this phase, we prepare your body for the cleanse. We want to begin to remove toxins, and to make sure your body is in an ideal state to receive all the benefits of the juices you'll be making in the juice-cleanse phase.

Do not skip this step! What you need to remember is that your body is adept at storing toxins in all of your cells. One of the purposes of the Juice Cleanse Reset Diet is to rid the body of those toxins. However, the detoxification process can have unpleasant side effects depending on the severity of toxins in your body. Just like in our imaginary office, as we pull out junk from its hiding places, things may look and feel worse before they get better. Jumping into the juice-cleanse phase cold turkey won't feel good, and it won't give you lasting results.

For example, if you haven't been eating organic produce and hormone-free meats or seafood, your hormones may be so out of balance that your food cravings are more closely tied to your emotions than to hunger. You'll need to reset your attitude and mindset and learn to understand when you're truly hungry or when you're facing some other issue and merely using food to divert your attention.

If you live on coffee, diet Coke, or energy drinks, your body is likely addicted to caffeine and your adrenal glands are overtaxed. You'll need to reset your energy level and metabolism. When cleansing, you may at first feel tired and sluggish without the chemicals your body has come to rely on.

If you rarely eat fruits and vegetables, your taste buds and sense of smell are probably so confused by chemicals and additives that real food may taste bland or "earthy" to you. You'll need to reset your taste buds to be able to taste all the deliciousness that Mother Nature has to offer.

If you've been consuming mostly processed food rather than whole grains, fruits, and veggies, you probably have stomachaches, indigestion, and trouble going to the bathroom. You'll need to reset your digestive system. You're so accustomed to feeling horrible after a meal, that you can't even remember what it's like to have no issues from food. You'll be amazed at how great you feel while on the Juice Cleanse Reset Diet!

If you've been struggling with your weight, feeling less beautiful than you would like, and cannot seem to stay away from fried food, sweets, snacks, and similar foods, you'll need to reset your weight, attitude, taste buds, and all the rest! Once you successfully rid your body of stored-up toxins and begin filling your body with organic fruits and vegetables, you'll be amazed at how the excess pounds melt off, your skin improves, and people begin commenting on how "rested," "youthful," and "glowing" you look!

WHAT TO EXPECT

Precleansing is the first step to resetting. Remember, by precleansing for a period of time, the body can begin removing those toxins because it will not be working as hard to remove and process toxins from the daily food intake. This will increase the efficacy of the juice cleanse itself, because the cells of the body will be better able to absorb all of the great nutrients and live enzymes contained in the juices. Think of this as removing the mess from our imaginary desk to make room for all the new filing systems and organization.

Through the precleanse phase, we'll slowly remove substances like caffeine, processed sugar, fatty foods, dairy, and meat so that the body can adjust to those changes and any withdrawal symptoms that may accompany them. Of course, if one eats a mainly vegetarian diet with few processed foods or added chemicals, the precleanse phase can be relatively short. For those who live on fast food and diet Coke, the process must be longer. As we discussed in the last chapter, the length of your precleanse phase depends on your current habits and choices. If you haven't yet taken the test to determine your type, go ahead and take it now (see page 42).

Type 1 cleansers will precleanse for two days.

Type 2 cleansers will precleanse for three days.

Type 3 cleansers will precleanse for four days.

Type 4 cleansers will precleanse for seven days.

No special equipment is needed for the precleanse. Any standard blender will suffice for the smoothies, and the meals are simple and plant based, using fresh ingredients you can easily find at the local grocery store or farmers' market (see chapter 2 for tips on shopping).

As we mentioned above, the precleanse phase will gradually reduce your consumption of meat, dairy, and processed food as you move toward your juice cleanse. It will also increase your daily intake of fruits and vegetables to increase the alkalinity in your body and begin resetting your taste buds. The all-liquid days flood your body with a bounty of alkaline fruits and veggies. Including more fresh and organic produce during the precleanse phase will help you avoid any negative side effects (headaches, nausea) that can happen when you transition from an acidic to an alkaline diet too quickly. Increasing the alkalinity of your body slowly will help you transition to the all-liquid portion of the cleanse with ease.

THE DOS AND DON'TS OF THE JUICE CLEANSE RESET DIET

As you embark on the precleanse phase, we'd like to share a few important components that will help ensure your success. We call these the dos and don'ts of the Juice Cleanse Reset Diet. Follow these components throughout the program, and you'll find they've become habit by the end of the program. If you continue with these practices daily, you'll maintain your reset results for the rest of your life.

Do Drink Water

Increase the amount of water you drink. Your body needs water to function properly, and water will also help wash away those toxins your body begins to release. Regardless of your type, begin each day with 16 ounces of room-temperature or warm water with lemon in it. This will get your digestive system and your metabolism moving. Throughout the rest of the day, continue to drink water at each meal for a total of at least 64 ounces per day. Beyond the 16 ounces of warm or room-temperature lemon water in the morning, we aren't super picky about what kind or temperature of water you drink, other than making sure it's well filtered. The most important thing is that you increase your water consumption. Drink it hot or cold, and feel free to add lemon or lime if you like. If you prefer carbonated water, you can drink that any time water is called for in the menu, unless you begin to notice abdominal discomfort, which may be attributable to the CO_2 in carbonated water. Bottled, filtered, or tap water all qualify, and you can certainly drink more than the amount prescribed. The amounts listed in the menu should be considered a minimum.

Don't Drink Caffeine

If you normally drink coffee, now is the time to wean yourself off of it. Coffee is acidic, and we're striving to restore alkalinity during the Juice Cleanse Reset Diet, so you'll be taking a break (at least for the length of the cleanse, if not longer) from coffee. If you aren't comfortable quitting cold turkey, limit yourself to one cup a day, and if you don't like it black, make yourself some homemade Almond Milk (page 181), and pour a little of that into your coffee.

Ideally, you'll replace your coffee with a caffeine-free green tea or other organic tea by the time you complete the precleanse phase. If you find that you are really struggling with giving up caffeine, you may drink caffeinated green tea (its health benefits outweigh the negative effects of the caffeine). Study after study has linked tea—green, black, oolong, and white—to an array of health benefits, including lower cholesterol, stronger bones, and lower rates of cardiovascular disease and cancer. Feel free to drink organic herbal tea as much as you wish during your Juice Cleanse Reset Diet. Don't use it as a substitute for water, however. You'll still need to drink your 64 ounces of water.

Do Buy Organic

As we discussed in the last chapter, it's very important that you choose organic whenever possible for many reasons, including the fact that nutrients in organic produce are superior to those in conventional produce. As we gradually increase your intake of fruits and veggies, we want to be sure you're getting the most nutrients available, without also increasing your ingestion of pesticides! If you can't afford to always buy organic, focus on the foods you eat most often and those that are most likely to be contaminated with pesticides. Refer to the Dirty Dozen chart (see page 28) that tells you the most important items to buy organic. Bring this book with you to the grocery store if you can't remember.

Although organic may be a bit more expensive than conventional, your body will thank you. You can also help keep those cost differences down by choosing fruits and veggies that are in season where you live, buying from the local farmers' market (a very easy way to find out what's growing locally at any time of year), or buying frozen. The freezing process generally does not harm the nutrients in fruits and vegetables, so it's a perfectly acceptable alternative to fresh. If, for instance, one of our recipes calls for blueberries, but you're reading this while a snowstorm rages outside, either buy frozen organic berries or choose an alternate recipe.

Don't Eat Meat and Poultry

Don't worry, we're not trying to turn you into a vegetarian (but we do want you to incorporate more fruits and veggies into your diet). Although we'll wean you off animal products in the precleanse phase, you'll be able to add them back in the postcleanse, to the extent that you want to. Some nutrients necessary for the proper functioning of the human body are much more readily available in animal products than in plants. Of course, whether you eat these things is a personal decision, but we want you to choose wisely if you do choose to eat meat, chicken, and eggs (as we discussed in the last chapter).

Do Choose Alkaline over Acidic Foods

If you've gone through life thinking that you're not a great multitasker, it turns out you were wrong! Your body automatically multitasks, regulating your temperature, blood sugar, vitamin D, and oxygen levels twenty-four hours a day. Another very important task that your body does automatically is regulate your acid/alkaline ratio.

pH Made Easy

More hydrogen = more acidity

More oxygen = more alkalinity

P stands for potency and H stands for hydrogen; pH stands for *potency of hydrogen*. More hydrogen equals greater alkalinity and more oxygen equals more acidity. Your body is designed to operate at a slightly alkaline state, with a blood pH just above 7. An overly acidic pH leads to inflammation, resulting in disease, illness, and fatigue. Since your body is hardworking and quite resourceful, it won't allow you to live in a dangerously acidic state. Instead, if your blood veers into an overly acidic state, the alkaline minerals from your tissues, organs, bones, and teeth will be drawn out in order to bring your pH back into balance. After your body uses these alkaline minerals to restore its desired pH, they are released from your body through urine. According to a 2011 study published by the *Journal of Environmental and Public Health*, the "quantity of calcium lost in the urine with the modern diet over time could be as high as 480 grams over twenty years or almost half the skeletal mass of calcium." No wonder there has been such an increase in bone density issues like osteoporosis. The moral of the story is: help yourself stay alkaline by eating your fruits and veggies!

Alkaline-Forming Foods

- Alkaline water

- Apple cider vinegar

- Avocados

- Citrus: lemon, lime, grapefruit

- Cold-pressed oils

- Grasses: wheat, barley

- Green tea

- Green veggies: spinach, kale, asparagus

- Fermented foods: sauerkraut, kimchi

- Miso

- Nuts: almonds, cashews

- Root vegetables: beet, sweet potato, turnip, jicama

- Seaweed

- Sprouts

- Stevia

Acid-Forming Foods

- Alcohol
- Animal protein: especially red meat
- Chemicals: all artificial additives
- Coffee
- Dairy

- Margarine
- Soda
- Soy
- White sugar
- Wheat
- Yeast
- Vinegar

Stress and all of its triggers—lack of sleep, emotions, living a sedentary lifestyle—lead to acidity. Your body constantly undergoes stresses that may contribute to acidity. You can decrease the detrimental impact of these stressors on your body by consuming a diet rich in alkaline foods, or you can exacerbate the problems by eating an acidic diet. Eating 100 percent alkaline foods is a lofty goal for even the most disciplined of eaters. The good news is that you don't have to consume 100 percent alkaline foods in order to increase your alkalinity. The precleanse phase is designed to shift your diet so that you're eating approximately 85 percent alkaline foods.

ACID TO ALKALINE

pH is quantified on a scale of 1 to 14; 7 is neutral.
Below 7 is acid and above 7 is alkaline.

pH=0	Hydrochloric acid (secreted from stomach lining)	DEMINERALIZATION
pH=1	Battery acid	
pH=2	Cola, vinegar	
pH=3	Apple, grapefruit juice	
pH=4	Beer, tomatoes, lemon-lime soda	
pH=5	Pickle juice, black coffee	
pH=6	Egg yolks, urine, skim milk, root beer	
pH=7	Human blood, wheatgrass	
pH=8	Seawater, chia seeds	REMINERALIZATION
pH=9	Baking soda	
pH=10	Household ammonia	
pH=11	Milk of magnesia	
pH=12	Soapy water	
pH=13	Lye, oven cleaner	
pH=14	Sodium hydroxide	

Not All Acids Are Bad

It's important to understand that some acids are natural. Your body efficiently deals with acids that are the by-products of respiration, metabolism, exercise, and cell turnover, and also produces one acid itself, called hydrochloric acid (HCl). HCl is essential to maintaining the proper acidity level in your gut for optimal digestion and to help protect you against potentially harmful bacteria that may be found in food.

Don't Wait to Plan Ahead

One of the key ingredients to sticking to the precleanse phase is proper planning. We suggest you go shopping on a weekend, and use our shopping list to purchase all of the items you'll need for the week. You can prepare some of the meals on Sunday, and then pack your meals and snacks each night for the next day. This way, you won't find yourself without food when you're out or at work. You'll use your meals, juices, and smoothies to get your body accustomed to burning calories throughout the day. Feel free to take shortcuts, like using organic canned beans (free from additives, of course) and prechopped vegetables or fruit. But we do want you to make the meals yourself rather than getting takeout from a restaurant, because that is the only way that you can truly know what ingredients go into your meals.

It's important that you choose a time for your cleanse when you have limited social or travel commitments. You'll find it much more difficult to stick to your days of structured meals and juices if you're attending a celebration on Saturday night. Planning your cleanse during an appropriate time sets you up for success. However, if you're not able to clear your social calendar, it doesn't mean you need to fall off the wagon. You can always choose a green salad with oil and vinegar or fresh lemon juice, a grilled vegetable plate, a broth-based vegetarian soup, or a fresh fruit plate if you're at a business or social engagement that requires you to participate in a meal. Drink plenty of water to help keep yourself full and avoid temptation, and then go back to the plan for your next meal. You don't need to announce that you're on a "special diet" because healthy food can be found on any menu if you know what to look for and are determined to succeed.

If you need to cook dinner and prepare meals for your family, put them on the same meal plan as you. All of the recipes are nutritious and delicious and creative enough to satisfy even the most picky eaters. If your family wants meat when you're on a vegetarian day, pick up an organic rotisserie chicken from the supermarket to supplement whatever you're making.

THE PRECLEANSE RESETS

During the precleanse phase, you'll begin resetting many areas of your health. Pay attention to these resets to recognize how the changes feel as they occur.

Reset Your Attitude and Your Mindset

You'll become conscious of what you put into your body, and make sure you have your healthy meals and snacks with you. It's easier to slip when you fail to plan or pay attention. Resetting your attitude and your mindset is intregal to your plan for success.

Reset Your Energy

If caffeine or energy drinks were a daily occurrence for you before the precleanse, you may find that your energy levels actually slump during this phase, as you eliminate these stimulants from your diet. Realize that this energy slump is only temporary; your energy will soar in just a few short days. Removing these items from your diet is important to the success of the Juice Cleanse Reset Diet and will make the juice-cleanse phase much more effective. If you need an energy boost to help you beat your slump, eat a piece of fruit, take a nap if possible, or go for a quick walk.

Reset Your Metabolism

By eating something every three hours or so, you'll get your metabolism burning more calories. You won't be skipping meals or snacks or feeling like you're famished at night, and you should be able to control those late-night munchies better.

Reset Your Taste Buds

During the precleanse phase, you'll eliminate all processed foods and increase your consumption of fruits and vegetables. Although vegetables may not taste great to you at first, as you remove the chemicals from your diet, your taste buds will begin to readjust.

Reset Your Digestive System

As you replace the processed food, dairy, fried food, meat, and so on with whole grains, fruits, and vegetables, you'll notice some changes in your digestion. Chances are that your bowel movements will become more regular and that you'll experience less digestive discomfort.

Reset Your Weight

Start paying attention to your weight and the way your clothes fit. If you want to lose weight, keep that goal at the forefront of your mind to help keep you strong through moments of temptation.

Reset Your Beauty

As you remove the processed food and alcohol from your diet and transition to real food, you'll notice a reduction in the bags under your eyes and puffiness in your face. Even small changes in what you put into your body affect your beauty.

THE PRECLEANSE MENUS

The daily meal plans below are a road map to make your journey easier. They set forth the path, but the driving is up to you. If you don't like something on the plan, feel free to swap out a meal with another recipe in the same section (see chapter 8 for recipes). Meals are organized into breakfast, lunch, dinner, and snacks. As long as you're choosing an alternate recipe from the same category, you'll stay on track. Of course, if you're a vegetarian or vegan, you'll substitute a vegan or vegetarian selection for any meal that includes dairy, meat, eggs, or fish. If you're an omnivore, no matter how much you love meat and dairy, it's very important that your meals on the day prior to starting the juice-cleanse phase *do not* include these items. Trust us—it will make the transition to juice easier.

Remember, the length of the precleanse is determined by the type of cleanser you are. If you're type 4, you'll start at seven days before the juice cleanse. If you're type 3, you'll start at four days before the juice cleanse. If you're type 2, you'll start at three days before the juice cleanse. And if you're type 1, you'll start at two days before the juice cleanse. Over the course of the precleanse days, you'll be changing your eating habits to a very alkaline, vegetarian diet. Regardless of type, everyone's final two days before the juice-cleanse phase will be the same.

You may be tempted to shorten the number of days you stay in the precleanse phase. Don't succumb to the temptation. This is a life journey to health, not a crash diet. The more closely you adhere to the plan, the greater your chance of lifetime success—and also the more pleasant the juice cleanse itself will be. Rushed detox is a fad and is not pleasant!

Seven Days Before the Juice Cleanse

Type 4 Cleansers

Upon Rising
16 ounces warm or room-temperature water, with lemon

Breakfast
16 ounces water
Roasted Vegetable Frittata (page 183)
2 slices whole-grain toast, dry

Lunch
16 ounces water
Turkey Patty (page 184)
Tomato-Avocado Salad (page 184)

Snack
16 ounces water
Handful of raw almonds
1 piece of fruit

Dinner
16 ounces water
Roasted Chicken (page 194)
Roasted Root Vegetables with Butternut Squash (page 207)
½ cup Cooked Quinoa (page 206)

Six Days Before the Juice Cleanse

Type 4 Cleansers

Upon Rising
16 ounces warm or room-temperature water, with lemon

Breakfast

16 ounces water
½ cup Steel-Cut Oatmeal (page 183)
3 scrambled egg whites
½ avocado

Lunch

16 ounces water
Spinach Salad (page 195)
Broiled Salmon (page 211)

Snack

16 ounces water
½ cup cooked and shelled edamame (soybeans)

Dinner

16 ounces water
Mixed Green Salad (page 198) with Balsamic Vinaigrette
   (page 230)
½ cup cooked whole wheat or gluten-free pasta, any type
½ cup Marinara Sauce (page 212)
1 Turkey Patty (page 194)

Five Days Before the Juice Cleanse

Type 4 Cleansers

Upon Rising

16 ounces warm or room-temperature water, with lemon

Breakfast

16 ounces water
Cucumber Watermelon Juice (page 187)
4 scrambled egg whites

Lunch

16 ounces water
Chicken Salad (page 200) on wheat bread

Snack

16 ounces water

½ cup plain Greek yogurt

½ cup mixed berries, such as strawberries, raspberries, or blueberries

Dinner

16 ounces water

Sautéed Spinach (page 227)

Pan-Seared Scallops (page 213)

½ cup Cooked Quinoa (page 221)

Four Days Before the Juice Cleanse

Type 3 and Type 4 Cleansers

Upon Rising

16 ounces warm or room-temperature water, with lemon

Breakfast

16 ounces water

Roasted Vegetable Frittata (page 183)

Lunch

16 ounces water

Spinach Salad (page 195)

Roasted Chicken Breast (page 208)

Snack

16 ounces water

2 Hard-Boiled Eggs Filled with Smashed Avocado (page 192)

Dinner

16 ounces water

Turkey-Stuffed Peppers (page 197)

Mixed Green Salad (page 188) with 2 tablespoons Lemon Vinaigrette (page 212)

Three Days Before the Juice Cleanse

Type 2, Type 3, and Type 4 Cleansers

Upon Rising
16 ounces warm or room-temperature water, with lemon

Breakfast
16 ounces water
Banana-Berry Smoothie (page 175)

Lunch
16 ounces water
Roasted Veggie and Chicken Salad (page 186)

Snack
16 ounces water
6 sticks celery
2 tablespoons Almond Butter (page 193)

Dinner
16 ounces water
Fish Baked in Foil (page 198)
Roasted Root Vegetables with Butternut Squash (page 207)

Two Days Before the Juice Cleanse

All Cleanser Types

Upon Rising
16 ounces warm or room-temperature water, with lemon

Breakfast
16 ounces water
Green Banana Smoothie (page 173)

Lunch
16 ounces water
Kale-Quinoa Salad (page 187)

Snack

16 ounces water

16 baby carrots with 2 tablespoons Hummus (page 191)

Dinner

16 ounces water

Veggie Stir-Fry with Brown Rice (page 201)

One Day Before the Juice Cleanse

All Cleanser Types

Upon Rising

16 ounces warm or room-temperature water, with lemon

Breakfast

16 ounces water

Green Banana Smoothie (page 173)

Lunch

16 ounces water

Simple Kale Salad (page 187)

Snack

16 ounces water

2 tablespoons Almond Butter (193)

1 small apple

Dinner

16 ounces water

Tomato-Vegetable Soup (page 204)

Listen to your body during this phase. You may go through some detox symptoms—like headaches, nausea, or sluggishness—before you feel more energized. You may find you crave processed food, caffeine, or sugar if they are part of your normal diet. If these cravings or other side effects haven't fully subsided by the last day before the juice cleanse, spend another day or two in the precleanse phase. The purpose is to prepare you properly to get the most out of your juice cleanse, so take your time preparing. The main goal is to enter the juice-cleanse phase having eaten a diet consisting mainly of fruits and veggies and no processed food.

Congratulations! You've made it through the first phase. Now that you have successfully removed processed food from your diet and begun consuming more alkaline foods, you should notice that you're feeling more energized. Whether you spent two or seven days precleansing, you should be craving more fruits and vegetables. The sludge is beginning to loosen itself from your cell walls.

At this point, your attitude toward food has probably changed somewhat. You are likely getting hungry every few hours, because you have been fueling your body with nutritious food regularly, and your metabolism is speeding up. If you didn't find "healthy" food tasty before now, we hope some of our recipes have changed your mind. Real food served simply has a lot of flavor, and your taste buds should be waking up to this realization now that the chemicals have been removed from your diet. Are you having fewer digestive issues—gas, indigestion, or heartburn? Your digestive system is starting to reset itself. You may even have started to lose weight or at least some of the puffiness and bloating in your body and face that hides your natural beauty. Take a moment to feel a sense of accomplishment on finishing your precleanse. Regardless of how long you spent in this phase, you did it, and you're now ready to begin your juice cleanse. Let's do it!

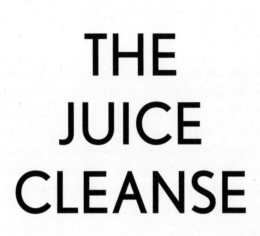

four

THE JUICE CLEANSE

"The best of all medicine is resting and fasting."

—Ben Franklin

Now that you have successfully prepared yourself, the next phase is juice! For the next three days, all of your meals will be liquid. (We'll discuss this in further detail later in the chapter, but if you don't have a juicer, don't worry. You can also cleanse by making smoothies in a blender. Your juice cleanse will just be lengthened to five days.) This phase is when you flood your body with nutrients. Do not think of it as deprivation; it's whole-food based, but you'll be drinking your meals instead of chewing.

THE JUICE CLEANSE RESETS

As with each part of the Juice Cleanse Reset Diet, the juice cleanse presents opportunities for you to reset many areas of your health, depending on your personal priorities. You may be wondering how you'll be able to tell whether you're successfully resetting. Here are some of the noticeable benefits:

- Abundance of energy and stamina
- Radiant skin
- Increased mental clarity
- Better sleep

- Empowered sense of self
- Happier mood
- Better digestion
- Decreased cravings for processed food
- Increased appetite for fruits and vegetables
- Feeling of lightness
- Leaner midsection
- Weight loss

You may experience all or only some of these benefits, and in some cases, the toxins leaving your body may make you feel a bit worse before you feel better. Here's what you can expect while you're resetting each area of your health.

Reset Your Attitude and Your Mindset

Your attitude will benefit from the mental clarity and sense of well-being derived from this juice cleanse. Abstaining from food, and saving the energy that goes into preparing and digesting meals, leads to a greater level of mindfulness. We encourage you to spend time during your juice cleanse reflecting on what food you put into your body and the effect it has inside and out. Juice cleansing is also the ideal way to reset your thought processes. You might be thinking you could never go one whole day without food, let alone three or five days, but you *can* do it. And we bet that your attitude about food will have changed by the time you finish this phase. While cleansing, you'll learn to recognize those times when you're craving food but not actually hungry. The juices will provide your body with all the nutrients it needs. You'll begin to understand that your cravings are generally related to emotional needs, boredom, stress, and social factors instead of hunger. You'll feel empowered to find that you can say no to those cravings.

Reset Your Energy

As you feed your body a steady stream of nutrients and it releases toxins, your energy level will rise. By consuming nutrient-dense drinks every couple of hours, your energy will actually increase over the course of the day, and you won't experience that midafternoon slump.

Reset Your Metabolism

Your energy is increasing because your metabolism is speeding up. As your body becomes accustomed to receiving nutritious fuel every couple of hours, you will begin burning fat rather than storing it.

Reset Your Taste Buds

Although you have weaned yourself off processed food and chemicals during the precleanse phase, you're now giving your body nothing but fruits and vegetables in large quantities. Because our bodies were designed to extract and use nutrients from the food we ingest, your body is going to be very happy to find itself inundated with organic nutrition. Once it gets a taste, it will crave more.

Reset Your Digestive System

For the next three days, you'll give your digestive system a complete break from its normal daily task of breaking down your food so that you can really absorb and use all the great nutrients that you crave. It takes approximately eighteen hours for your body to eliminate one meal. If you normally eat three meals a day, your digestive system is working around the clock! With a diet of liquids for three days, your digestive system gets to rest, focus on removing toxins, and heal itself. At the same time, the juices will flood your body with live enzymes, nutrients, and vitamins, further speeding the detoxification and healing processes. Digestive problems, such as chronic bloat and discomfort, will be all but a memory. Juice cleansing is an optimal way to give your body a break while feeding it all the nutrients it needs. If you are using a blender to make smoothies, your digestive system won't completely shut down, but you will be making the job of digestion much easier by blending your food into smoothies.

Reset Your Weight

Although the reason for doing a cleanse is not to lose weight, you'll be pleased to notice that you're dropping excess pounds during your cleanse and afterward. As your body releases toxins, your abdomen will become leaner and less bloated. Your healthier cravings will help you continue to lose or maintain your perfect weight after the cleanse, too.

Reset Your Beauty

You wash your face and body every day, probably more than once. You moisturize with expensive products and creams, but from a beauty perspective, cleaning your insides is even more important than caring for the outside. Those built-up toxins from the environment and food will clog your pores and make your skin dull, your hair limp, and your face puffy. By removing those toxins and filling your body with nutrients, your beauty will also increase. Over time, your nails will be stronger, your hair thicker, and your complexion clearer. The radiance will shine through!

DETOX SYMPTOMS

During the juice-cleanse phase of the diet, you may experience some detox symptoms. If you do experience symptoms (some people call this a "healing crisis"), it may be a sign that your cells are releasing toxins more quickly than they are being eliminated. Detox symptoms display themselves differently for each person, but they may include headaches, fatigue, nausea, rashes, or temporary bloating. While your body is capable of working through this on its own, the more you do to assist your body in the elimination of these toxins, the more quickly the symptoms will dissipate. Here are some ideas that will help you deal with any detox symptoms that come up.

Have a Dry Brush

Dry brushing, which opens up your pores for toxin elimination, is one of the easiest, least expensive, and most effective things you can do to improve your skin. Try to do this daily before showering or bathing to increase the benefits of your reset and improve the quality, tone, and texture of your skin. Dry brushing stimulates the lymphatic system to release toxins and mobilizes fat cells by breaking up toxic deposits of stored fatty tissue (aka cellulite). Consistent dry brushing reveals healthier, smoother, more youthful-looking skin.

Use a natural (nonsynthetic) brush, with stiff yet nonabrasive bristles. Make long sweeps starting at your feet and moving up the legs toward your heart. Next, from there, brush from the arms toward your chest. Avoid circular, back and forth or scrubbing motions. On your stomach, move the brush in a counterclockwise movement. Be careful not to brush too hard. Your goal is to stimulate your skin without causing irritation.

Enjoy a Sauna Session

Spending time in a sauna is a relaxing way to wake up your cleansing organs, work up a sweat, and burn extra calories. Because your skin is your biggest organ of elimination, breaking a sweat is a great way to eliminate toxins. Infrared saunas, which generate heat on a cellular level, are our first pick. If you don't have access to an infrared, any sauna will be beneficial!

Be sure to consume lots of water on days that you use the sauna. Consuming water helps replenish your electrolyte levels and keeps your body in balance. For an extra energy boost, try immediately following your sauna session with a cold shower.

Take a Detox Bath

If you don't have access to a sauna, a detox bath is fantastic alternative that gives you equal results. Soaking in a sweat-inducing detox bath is a surefire way to quickly release impurities and acidic waste through your skin. Combine 2 cups of Epsom salts, 1 cup of baking soda, and a few bags of ginger tea or 2 tablespoons of ground ginger to a warm bath. You may also consider adding 1 cup of apple cider vinegar. Soak for 20 to 30 minutes.

Drink Herbal Teas

Consuming only cold beverages lowers your core body temperature and your body has to expend extra energy to keep warm. Adding herbal teas will help regulate your temperature and also provide the added benefit of supporting your detox with herbs. Herbal teas containing milk thistle, lemongrass, or dandelion root help support your liver in flushing toxins out of your body. Mint, anise, and ginger all soothe your stomach. Herbal teas containing senna or cascara sagrada are plant-based laxatives that will encourage elimination to push toxins through and out.

Do a Colonic

If you're suffering from a "healing crisis," you may want to consider a colonic in order to remove toxins quickly. Colon hydrotherapy is a gentle, odorless, and clean process in which water flows gently into your colon via a tube. When the water is released, it carries accumulated waste out with it. The process is controlled by a certified colon hydrotherapist.

WHAT TO EXPECT

After years of counseling clients through our three-day juice cleanse, we've come to recognize commonalities in the way the cleanse affects people. It may vary by the day, but by day 3 you should be experiencing most of the benefits mentioned below.

Day 1

You'll begin your day with a glass of warm or room-temperature water with some fresh lemon squeezed into it. This is a habit you began during the precleanse phase, and one that you should maintain throughout the juice cleanse and for the rest of your life. You also increased your water consumption in the precleanse; you should continue this while on the juice cleanse, too. Drinking water between juices will help flush out the toxins. Do not skip drinking water; this is just as important as the juices.

On the first day of the cleanse, the green juices may take some getting used to, especially if you're accustomed to drinking sugary beverages or pasteurized juices. Choose the recipes with more fruit if you're having a hard time with the green juices at first. You may also feel like there are a *lot* of juices to drink. Try to be really disciplined about drinking a juice every two hours, even if you aren't hungry yet. You want to keep your body consistently fueled so it becomes accustomed to burning calories constantly throughout the day. Also, if you skip a few juices and wait until you're ravenous before drinking one, they won't be as satisfying as when you stick to a schedule.

If you can't get through all six juices, that's okay, but even if you skip one or two, be sure to end your day with one of the nut milks. If you're allergic to nuts, drink the hemp milk because it has the same benefits. Because the juice cleanse is calorie restrictive, a high-protein, higher fat juice (like one made with nuts or hemp) at night will be very important to helping you sleep well.

If you were really strict during the precleanse phase, you'll likely be feeling great. If you had trouble kicking caffeine, or sneaked in a few processed foods, you may experience a dull headache, feel a little nauseated, or lack energy. These symptoms are perfectly normal. You're removing the toxins from their hiding places in your cells and organs, and as they pass through the body on their way out, they may leave some unpleasant feelings.

You may feel hungry, as your digestive system is used to working and now doesn't have much substance to break down. And you may feel unsatisfied because you're used to chewing and you haven't had the pleasure of chewing solid food. If you truly feel like you need solid food, it is completely okay to honor that feeling. Have a small piece of organic fruit, some cucumber slices, or half an avocado with fresh lemon. Eat mindfully, paying attention to how the food satisfies your hunger. Drink water after eating and then continue on with your liquid program.

Alternatively, you may feel super full from all the juice and water, especially if you don't normally drink many fluids during the day. You may also be going to the bathroom every hour (number 1, not number 2!) because of all the liquids. That may be time-consuming, but it means your body is ridding itself of toxins, so embrace it.

You may find that you have lots of energy in the afternoon, or you may feel like you want a nap. If you're able to nap, go for it. If not, and you feel you need energy, take a brisk walk for ten minutes.

If you feel bored because your evening isn't taken up by preparing and eating food, use that time to reflect on what you have accomplished and to practice gratitude about all the positive things and people in your life. You could also use the time to go for a walk or to the gym. Movement will help speed the detox process.

Day 2

On the second day, you'll probably wake up feeling rested because you had such a great night's sleep. You'll also feel a little lighter and possibly light-headed. If you didn't feel hungry or tired yesterday, chances are that you will today. Take a nap if you feel like it. Go to the gym and get energized by that amazing spin teacher. Eat half an avocado with a spoon if you need to, and savor it as if it's a bowl of ice cream. Congratulate yourself on being more than halfway through the juice cleanse.

MARY S., ATTORNEY • Mary wrote to us to tell us that one of the reasons she keeps doing our juice cleanse is because she sleeps so well, "like a little kid!" Normally, she has a terrible time sleeping. She wrote: "I have to think amazing things are happening and healing in my body to get me to sleep like that." Mary is right. Her body is able to use all that energy normally devoted to digesting food to repair her body. Because her digestive system is able to take a break, Mary is achieving a deep state of relaxation during her sleeping hours. Normally, her body is still busy breaking down food while she is sleeping. Now, she is completely in rest-and-repair mode during sleep. "I wake up feeling refreshed and ready to jump out of bed. This is a major change from my normal habit of hitting the snooze button three times before dragging myself to the kitchen where I make my morning coffee. Ambien would go out of business if everyone started juicing."

Day 3

You'll again wake up refreshed from your great night's sleep, and should also be feeling proud of yourself for making it this far. You'll either be counting down your juices in anticipation of solid food tomorrow, or more likely you'll be seriously considering extending the cleanse for a few more days. If you want to extend, you should definitely do it. In the first three days, there is a gentle release of toxins that restores balance to your system. On longer cleanses, you begin to repair your body on a cellular level, which helps you achieve a state of optimal well-being.

Regardless of whether you continue on for a few more days or move to the postcleanse phase, you have succeeded in resetting your attitude and mindset, energy level, metabolism, taste buds, digestive system, beauty, and perhaps weight. Those changes will be further reinforced during your postcleanse.

JUICE OR SMOOTHIE? JUICER OR BLENDER?

In order to start your juice cleanse, you'll need either a juicer or a blender. Juices are made in a juicer and smoothies are made in a blender. If you use a juicer, it will remove all or most of the fiber from your produce, leaving you with only the liquid nutrients. This is the preferred method for the cleanse, as it will be the fastest route to giving your digestive system a break.

If you don't have a juicer and aren't ready to purchase one, never fear. You can make smoothies in your blender, and still give your body the benefit of all those yummy little nutrients and enzymes contained in fruits and veggies. The only difference is that the smoothies still contain fiber.

You may be wondering, "Don't I need fiber in my diet? That's what my doctor is always telling me." Yes, in general you do need fiber to help your digestive system keep moving along. However, in the case of a juice cleanse, we're looking to give your digestive system a little vacation. By removing the fiber, the vacation starts right away, like being on a remote island with no cell phone and no email. You begin to chill out immediately. By using smoothies, it's like being out of the office but still connected to your computer; it takes a few more days to really feel relaxed. If you use a juicer, your juice cleanse will last three days. If you use a blender, you should stay on the juice cleanse for five days.

If you've decided to go the smoothie route, any blender will suffice, but the stronger the motor, the smaller the pulp will be and thus the more palatable the green smoothies will be.

Vitamix and Blendtec are the most common commercial blender brands. If you have either of these, all of the smoothie recipes will be easy for your blender, and your smoothies will have a fairly smooth consistency. If you have other household types of blenders, you may find you need to add more liquid to your smoothie to get it to a drinkable consistency, because the blender may not completely liquefy some of the fruit or the ice. You can add water, homemade almond or hemp milk, or coconut water.

If you choose to buy a juicer, you need to know that there are four main types, and you can feel comfortable in choosing whichever suits your needs and pocketbook best.

Centrifugal Juicer

The most common type of juicer is a centrifugal juicer. This is the type you see at your local juice bar, or may remember seeing Jack LaLanne use on his infomercials. With this type of juicer, you feed the fruits and vegetables through a chute, where they come into contact with a shredder disk with sharp blades that spins at high speeds while grinding and grating the fruits and vegetables into tiny pieces. The centrifugal force generated by the high-speed revolution pushes the juice through a fine-screen sieve, separating the pulp from the juice and depositing each into a separate container.

The pros:

- Juicer is less expensive than other juicers, typically between $90 and $220.

- It juices very quickly.

The cons:

- Cleanup is not easy.

- The juicer introduces a lot of oxygen into the juice while grinding and grating, resulting in juices that are only fresh for about twenty-four hours before the nutrients begin to die from exposure to oxygen.

- High-speed revolution causes heat and friction, which will begin to break down the nutrients and enzymes.

- Because centrifugal juicers move so quickly, the nutritional yield is lower than other methods. Some of the nutrients are left behind in the pulp.

Recommended centrifugal juicer models:

- Omega Big Mouth Juicer

- Breville Juice Fountain Elite

- Jack LaLanne's Power Juicer

- Omega 1000 Juicer

Masticating (Single Gear) Juicer

Masticating juicers "chew" the fruits and veggies to extract juice. They use a single gear, an auger with blades (teeth), to grind or crunch the vegetable and fruit fiber, slowly breaking up the cells.

The pros:

- The slower juicing process results in more vitamins, enzymes, and trace minerals contained in the juice. The slower rate of rotation generates less heat and injects less oxygen into the end product, protecting the nutrients in the juice and providing you with a healthier juice.

- Higher yield requires less produce.

- These juicers fall into the mid-range of cost, priced between $170 and $240.

The cons:

- Cleanup is more difficult and time-consuming than centrifugal juicers.
- Juicers are heavier (10 to 15 pounds), so they are not as portable.
- They aren't as good at juicing fruits and carrots.

Recommended masticating juicers:

- Omega J8006 Nutrition Center Juicer
- Oscar VitalMax 900 Cold-Press Juicer
- Champion Juicer

Triturating (Twin Gear) Juicer

This type of juicer uses two stainless steel twin gears to squeeze and press fruits and vegetables. It operates at very slow speeds, so nutrient value is high. The twin gears are very effective at squeezing the pulp, and produce a high yield of juice.

The pros:

- This type produces less foam and higher yield.
- The very slow speed extracts more nutrients and exposes ingredients to very little heat or oxygen.
- Juicer is quiet to operate.
- It's excellent for juicing leafy vegetables.
- Juicer is better than centrifugal juicers at juicing leafy greens.

The cons:

- Juicer is expensive, priced between $500 and $1,000.
- Juicing is slow and time-consuming.

Recommended twin gear juicers:

- Green Star Elite GSE-5000 Juicer
- Super Angel Juicer

Cold Pressed: Norwalk Juicer

The design and manufacturing of the Norwalk Juicer was prompted by Dr. Norman Walker, who is renowned for his research on the healthy benefits of eating raw food and drinking freshly made vegetable and fruit juices. The current model was developed in 1934. It's essentially a combination of two machines, a grinder and a hydraulic press. The grinder first crushes and grinds the produce into tiny pieces inside linen bags. The hydraulic press then extracts almost all of the juice by applying pressure from two stainless steel plates onto the linen bags.

The pros:

- This juicer extracts the highest percentage of juice.
- It makes foam-free juice with the lowest levels of oxidation.
- It produces juice with a long shelf life—juice will last in the fridge for two to three days.
- Juice has high nutrient density (four to seven times more than other juicers).
- Juice is pulpfree.

The cons:

- Juicer is expensive—$2,400.
- It is a heavy appliance, weighing nearly 50 pounds.

LET THE CLEANSE BEGIN

For the next three days (or five days, if you are using a blender) you'll reset your body by flooding it with nutrients. Think of this time as a vacation from chewing. You'll be feeding your body an abundance of healthy, nutritious juices. Once you get out of your head and begin listening to your body, you'll find the juices immensely satiating, and your body will thank you.

Each day of the cleanse should include six (16-ounce) juices, with a minimum of two greens, one nut milk, and one alkalizer. We have provided several recipes in each category, and the recipes include readily available vegetables and fruits. Because enzymes and nutrients are not significantly damaged by freezing, frozen fruit can also be used if fresh fruit cannot be easily obtained. Those allergic or sensitive to nuts can use protein substitutes like tofu and hemp milk. If you don't like an ingredient in a particular recipe, leave it out or substitute something else. Feel free to mix and match differently each day, or to stick to the same menu all three days. This is your cleanse, so do what feels comfortable for you.

Please choose organic ingredients whenever possible. Remember, the purpose of the cleanse is to rid your body of toxins, not load it up with more. Also, you want the most nutrient- and antioxidant-dense ingredients you can find because the juices are your food for the next three or more days.

Also, please do not buy juice from your supermarket in an effort to save time. That juice is pasteurized to extend shelf life, which means it has been heated to 140°F. In the process, many of the live enzymes have been destroyed. We want you to feed your body live fruits and veggies so you're energized and reset.

Freezing Herbs

If you love to add herbs like parsley or cilantro to your juices and smoothies, you have probably bought a whole big bunch and then only used a few sprigs. To use the whole bunch, put it in a food processor or blender and pulse the herbs with a little coconut oil. If you want, you can add some lemon juice to preserve the color. Place the chopped herbs in ice cube trays in the portion you would typically use for a smoothie or juice, add water, and freeze. Once frozen, add your herb cubes to a freezer-safe container or bag and use as needed.

THE JUICE CLEANSE SCHEDULE

You can make your nut milks once in a triple batch, and then store each serving in a 16-ounce mason jar, filled to the top and capped. Open a new one each evening. Juices and smoothies can be made each morning, placed in a mason jar with a cap, and consumed throughout the day. Recipes for juices and smoothies start on page 165.

You should drink the juices approximately two hours apart and finish the last one two hours prior to bedtime. Be sure to drink plenty of water or organic tea in between the juices to help flush toxins.

Upon Rising
16 ounces warm or room-temperature water
with lemon and a pinch of cayenne pepper (optional)

Meal One
Green juice or green smoothie

Meal Two
Fruit juice or fruit smoothie

Meal Three
Green juice or green smoothie

Meal Four
Alkalizer

Meal Five
Green juice or green smoothie

Meal Six
Nut milk or hemp milk

If you normally work out each day, continue to do so. If you normally do not, start now. Even a twenty-minute walk is going to help. Movement is important to the cleansing process; it helps all the toxins make their way out of the body. Choose a juice with some fruit in it prior to your workout. If your workout is strenuous, feel free to drink an extra juice or two that day. We recommend having an extra fruit juice before your workout for fuel and an extra nut milk after you train for recovery.

FOCUS ON YOUR RESETS

As you recall, you began the reset process in your precleanse phase. You may have noticed extreme resets, or you may have experienced only slight changes. During the juice cleanse, you'll really begin to see and feel the effects!

Reset Your Attitude and Your Mindset

Focus on the positive and on the language you use with yourself. Congratulate yourself for drinking your juice and going for a walk. Don't get down on yourself if you cheat and have a piece of fruit or a handful of nuts. You need to listen to your body, and if having a small apple makes it easier for you to stick to this cleanse, then go ahead.

We find that there are a few "cheat" foods that don't significantly reduce the effectiveness of the juice cleanse, but they can be satiating and take the edge off your hunger if you're struggling. Half an avocado with freshly squeezed lemon juice, some cucumber slices, a cup of vegetable broth, or a handful of raw almonds are acceptable.

Reset Your Energy

Feel how satisfying the juices are to your body. Enjoy the increased energy you experience as the day progresses. If you feel sluggish and tired, or achy and irritable, you're experiencing detox symptoms. Take a nap if possible, or go for a brisk walk and drink plenty of water. As toxins loosen from your cells, they'll pass through your body and can cause feelings of fatigue or nausea. Drinking water and moving will help those toxins leave your body more quickly, so you, too, will soon feel energized from your juices!

Reset Your Metabolism

You may notice that your body actually tells you when it's time for your next juice. As your metabolism increases and stabilizes, your body will burn fuel more efficiently. Don't skip juices, even if you don't feel hungry yet. Sticking to your schedule of a juice at least every two hours is important.

Reset Your Taste Buds

Try different recipes and ingredients. As you continue to drink your juices each day, pay attention to how much your body craves the nutrients and flavors of each. Notice how much sweeter the juices taste on day 3 than on day 1. You may be surprised to discover that you crave fruits and vegetables, even if you normally don't eat many. If you're tempted to eat some solid food, you're probably craving a strawberry more than a cupcake!

Reset Your Digestive System

Notice the way your digestive system starts to wake up with that first glass of warm lemon water. You may feel some rumbling in your tummy, or even find you're hungry even though you normally never eat breakfast. You may also find that your bowel movements are more regular. Stay on track by drinking a juice at least every two hours.

Reset Your Weight

As your metabolism increases and your body realizes it can count on receiving nutrients every two hours or so, you'll require more fuel and begin burning excess fat. You may first notice that your abdomen is flatter and tighter. If you feel bloated instead, that is a sign of detox. If you don't regularly take probiotics, now is the time to start. See chapter 6 for more information on probiotics and digestive enzymes.

Reset Your Beauty

Revel in the amazing sleep you get each night, and how much more rested you feel. Notice the changes in your skin and your eyes. Watch the puffiness under your eyes virtually disappear as your eyes become whiter and brighter. As the toxins leave your body and you continue to feed your body valuable enzymes and nutrients, your beauty will actually be rejuvenated, and your friends and family will notice!

You did it! Whether the past three days (or possibly more for you) were a breeze, the hardest thing you have ever done, or somewhere in between, you did it! Stop to congratulate yourself and reflect on all you have accomplished. You have cleaned out the gunk, and flooded your body with enzymes, antioxidants, vitamins, and minerals. You have reduced your toxic load, upped your nutrient intake, and reset your body. Notice your increased energy level, renewed taste buds, revved-up metabolism, rejuvenated beauty, new body weight, and, most importantly, your new and improved attitude toward food.

It's important that you tune in to all of your accomplishments. When you first picked up this book, you probably thought a juice fast was impossible, but here you are! You're well on your way to locking in new habits that will bring you greater long-term health.

During the next two days, we'll slowly wake up your digestive system by reintroducing solid food. The choices you make over the next few days will be important to the continuation of the success you've experienced. Use that positive attitude, your renewed energy, and your healthier cravings to continue to lose weight, rejuvenate your beauty, and embrace a healthier lifestyle. Let's get you chewing!

five

THE POST-CLEANSE PHASE

"Whether you think you can, or think you can't, you're right."

—Henry Ford

Congratulations on completing the liquid portion of your Juice Cleanse Reset Diet. Today you get to chew! Your full-body reset is well on its way. As you integrate whole food back into your diet, now is the perfect time to expand your reset to the rest of your life and lock in your new habits, cravings, and thoughts.

You exercised restraint and discipline during the juice cleanse. You were able to recognize the difference between being truly hungry and having emotional cravings for food. Successfully completing the juice-cleanse phase is an empowering experience worthy of celebration, even if you slipped up a few times. Remember that as you move forward, you have the power to choose your attitude, and your attitude strongly influences your results—so choose an attitude of success! Move past your slipups (there will be some) without judgment and reset your life one choice at a time.

If you understand the effects of each choice you make, and you're armed with the right tools (think back to the knowledge you gained in chapter 2 about how to decipher food labels and how to spot high-quality food sources), you're well prepared to make the best choices in any situation. If you're floating on cloud nine and feeling great, but you also find yourself having anxiety over reintroducing solid food, try to let go of that fear.

ATHANA H., SCHOOL ADMISSIONS DIRECTOR • I began my first Juice Cleanse Reset Diet about a year and a half ago. I had never tried a cleanse before, but I was fed up with myself and ready to make a change. As I neared my eighteenth wedding anniversary, I realized that the pound or two I'd gained each year since my wedding day had accumulated to a twenty-pound weight gain. I hadn't exercised in years and while I didn't eat poorly, I didn't give food much thought either. I felt sluggish and drained and looked tired. Over the past two decades, I had focused on taking care of my husband, raising our daughter, and working a full-time job; I had lost sight of prioritizing myself.

My goal in embarking on the seven-day program was to hit the reset button. I was hoping that I would have more energy at the end and more clarity and focus to start making better choices. And I did find that I was more energized than I had been in years. But I was surprised to also lose six pounds; friends and coworkers commented on my glowing skin and rested looks. People asked me if I'd been on vacation or had a little work done! That was the "aha" moment for me. I decided I didn't want to go backward from here, only forward. I wanted to turn that six-pound weight loss into twenty pounds, and I wanted to start taking care of myself again. I followed the program and integrated juices and smoothies into my day-to-day routine. I joined a local boot camp and now work out three days a week. Within six months, I had reached my goal weight and I have maintained that weight for over a year now.

Sometimes I get into a rut, make bad decisions, and gain a couple of pounds, but I know I can go back to the Juice Cleanse Reset Diet to get right back on track.

Athana's story is not unique. She took the resets she experienced from the juice cleanse and turned them into a reset lifestyle. The same can happen for you!

THE POSTCLEANSE RESETS

Taking moments during your day to reflect and be in touch with your body will keep you on track with your healthy habits and help you identify the foods that best feed your individual needs. Moving forward, pay attention to how food influences the reset areas:

Your attitude and your mindset: Do certain foods influence your mood?

Your energy: Do some foods give you energy, while others make you feel lethargic?

Your metabolism: Are you hungrier after consuming certain foods than others?

Your taste buds: Do you crave sugar or salt after consuming some types of food?

Your digestion: Do you have stomach discomfort after eating any meals?

Your weight: Do certain foods cause you to feel bloated?

Your beauty: Are any of the meals causing breakouts, rashes, or puffiness?

Reset Your Attitude and Your Mindset

Now that you have successfully made it three days without chewing, you know you can do anything you put your mind to! Forget those sugary cupcakes—a nice ripe peach should sound delicious at this point. You should feel empowered with the knowledge that you can control your eating.

Reset Your Energy

Without the huge job of digestion, your body has been able to reserve significant energy for the past three days. As you reintroduce food, make sure it's food that is full of enzymes and nutrients, real food that your body can use for energy rather than fake food that will zap your body of energy. The meal plan and recipes below will get you on the right track.

Reset Your Metabolism

You have taught your metabolism to expect nutrition every couple of hours on the juice cleanse. Nearly every calorie you took in was usable to your body. As you reintroduce solid food, you want to keep your metabolism running at high speed, by eating frequently and making sure the food you ingest is as nutritious as possible—no processed food!

Reset Your Taste Buds

All those delicious juices and smoothies reminded your taste buds how great real food tastes, and all those vitamins and nutrients reminded your cells that they thrive on nutrients. Listen to your taste buds and cravings. Do not go out and have a steak and martini dinner to celebrate eating solid food when your body tells you it wants fruits and veggies. The postcleanse will help you make the transition from juice to food easily and successfully.

Reset Your Digestive System

Your digestive system has had a nice three-day vacation. If you ask it to do something difficult right away, it won't be happy and it'll let you know. The postcleanse menu will transition you from juice to solid food in a way that will be easiest on your digestive system.

Reset Your Weight

Because you have removed toxins and reset your cravings, your healthy choices over the next few days should lead to more weight loss, if you are overweight. Many of our clients experience more weight loss in the few days that follow the juice cleanse than they did during the liquid portion of the diet.

Reset Your Beauty

Now that you have started to repair your skin cells and remove all the excess toxins, your skin looks great. The food you eat on the post-cleanse will be alkalizing, nutrient dense, and full of live enzymes, and you'll continue to see improvements in the way you look.

IDENTIFY TRIGGER FOODS

In addition to flooding your body with vital nutrients and enzymes, part of what makes the Juice Cleanse Reset Diet effective is what you *aren't* consuming. Many people go through life with undetected allergies or sensitivities to very common foods. They never knew how badly they felt until they feel good for the first time. If you have already seen an otherwise chronic rash disappear, mucus and sinus issues decrease, digestion issues go away, a major increase in your energy levels, or other substantial positive side effects from the cleanse, you could be one of these people with previously unidentified food sensitivities.

Upon successfully completing the precleanse and juice cleanse, your system is clear of the primary potential trigger foods, giving you the unique opportunity to start with a clean slate. If you suspect that you have food sensitivities, we suggest that you slowly and systematically reintroduce common trigger foods into your diet in order to monitor your body's reaction. Effectively identifying a trigger food could mean the difference between boundless energy and long-term weight-loss success or depleted energy combined with a host of other health concerns, including long-term weight struggles.

WILLIAM D., EMERGENCY ROOM DOCTOR • I became a juicing addict after my very first experience with the Juice Cleanse Reset Diet. I started doing a three-day cleanse every month religiously. Each time, I felt incredible and by day 3, I would be trimmer, I could breathe better, and my digestion was better. The results were always awesome. The only problem was that within one week of coming off of cleansing, my sinuses would get stuffed up again, the weight would come back, and my usual GI issues would return. I was frustrated and turned to Lori and Marra for some advice on how to extend the benefits I felt during the cleanses into my normal life. We went over the concept of food sensitivities, and we worked on gradually adding in foods like wheat, dairy, and soy after my cleanse. After following the protocol to add these foods in gradually, it was obvious that I had a major sensitivity to wheat! Now, having removed wheat from my diet completely, I'm feeling better than ever. I still love how I feel when cleansing, but I can do it less frequently now and maintain the same benefits.

The seven most common trigger foods are dairy, sugar/artificial sweeteners, soy, corn, gluten, eggs, and peanuts. Here's how to gradually reintroduce these potential trigger foods back into your diet:

1. Add only one trigger food at a time to isolate the cause of malaise.

2. Consume the trigger food two days in a row or twice in one day to get a good read if it is the culprit.

3. Wait a minimum of four days before adding another trigger food to allow your body adequate time in between to reset.

4. Add the purest form of the food back first. For example, if you are introducing wheat for the first time postcleanse, opt for sprouted whole grain bread rather than a bagel. If you add a processed form, you may experience a negative reaction to the preservatives or additives and mistake it for sensitivity to that food. Plus—you're not adding back processed foods *ever*, right?!

After completing the postcleanse menu plan below, you'll be responsible for planning your own meals again. Follow the steps above for gradual reintroduction of your potential trigger foods. If you feel fatigued, get a rash, experience bloating, or have other negative symptoms after adding dairy, sugar, soy, corn, gluten, eggs, or peanuts back into your diet, it's a good indicator that you have a sensitivity to this food. Once you identify sensitivity to a certain food, we recommend that you completely avoid this food for ninety days before experimenting with adding it back to your meals. After taking a complete break from the offending food for some time, you may be able to add moderate amounts of the food back into your diet without any negative effects. Listen to your body and determine this for yourself based upon how you feel. Enjoy following the postcleanse recipes and remember the rules for gradual inclusion once you venture into creating your own meal plans.

THE POSTCLEANSE PHASE

As you integrate whole food back into your diet, you need to be mindful that your digestive system has been shut down for the past three days. During the postcleanse, you'll slowly add different types of solid food to your diet, beginning with the easiest to digest. That means starting with fruits and vegetables, adding legumes, and then eventually animal protein, beginning with seafood and eggs because they are easiest to digest. If you're a vegetarian, or if you find that you just don't have a taste for animal protein right now, continue with plant-based food. What you definitely want to avoid during the next two days is eating red meat, dairy, greasy foods, and alcohol. None of these will make you feel good. It would be surprising if you crave any of those things, but if you are, use your new willpower to choose not to eat them for two more days.

Listen to your body! Be mindful of how each new item feels to you. If you don't want to eat dairy, or meat, or gluten, or soy, you don't need to. If there is any recipe below that doesn't appeal to your newly reset cravings and taste buds, feel free to substitute from the same category in the precleanse and postcleanse recipe sections. For instance, if you don't want to eat eggs for breakfast, go ahead and find another breakfast meal that sounds better, or stick with delicious smoothies every morning, if that feels better to your body.

If you're feeling scared of "undoing" all the resets when you start eating solid food, know that this postcleanse phase is designed to help you succeed. After all you have accomplished, we want to help you move forward with lifelong habits and changes. We also want to make sure your transition to solid food is pleasant and easy, as we get your digestive system operating again after its three-day sabbatical. Now that you know the types of food you'll be eating and why, let's get you chewing!

Day 1

Upon Rising
16 ounces warm or room-temperature water, with lemon

Breakfast
16 ounces water
Kiwi Berry Smoothie (page 177)

Lunch
16 ounces water
Mixed Green Salad (page 188) with vinaigrette of choice

Snack

16 ounces water

2 tablespoons Hummus (page 191)

16 baby carrots

Dinner

16 ounces water

Raw Red Pepper Soup (page 206)

Simple Kale Salad (page 187)

Day 2

Upon Rising

16 ounces warm or room-temperature water, with lemon

Breakfast

16 ounces water

Pineapple Banana Smoothie (page 178)

Lunch

16 ounces water

Mediterranean Salad (page 186)

Snack

16 ounces water

1 tablespoon Almond Butter (page 193)

1 apple

Dinner

16 ounces water

Shrimp Stir-Fry (page 201, variation)

½ cup cooked brown rice

If you want to continue on with the postcleanse portion of the Juice Cleanse Reset Diet for a bit longer, you can follow the precleanse recipes back out from your cleanse (see page 63). In other words, on day 3, follow the menu for Three Days Before the Juice Cleanse and on day 4, follow the menu for Four Days Before the Juice Cleanse, and so on. We have found that some people who feel great after the seven-day program are afraid to "mess it up" by eating the wrong things. By following the diet plan for five more days (by following the menus provided up to Seven Days Before the Juice Cleanse), your body will become so accustomed to healthy choices that your healthier cravings combined with your new mindful attitude will guide you in the right direction.

If you have completed the two postcleanse days and are ready to make your own meal choices, you're finished with the Juice Cleanse Reset Diet. Congratulations! Regardless of whether you're moving into the maintenance phase today, or in a couple of days, you don't need to be afraid. Making the right choices is simple once you have the tools. In the next chapter, we'll give you the knowledge about food and exercise to convert everything you've accomplished and learned over the past week into a reset lifestyle. Let's get you started on the rest of your life.

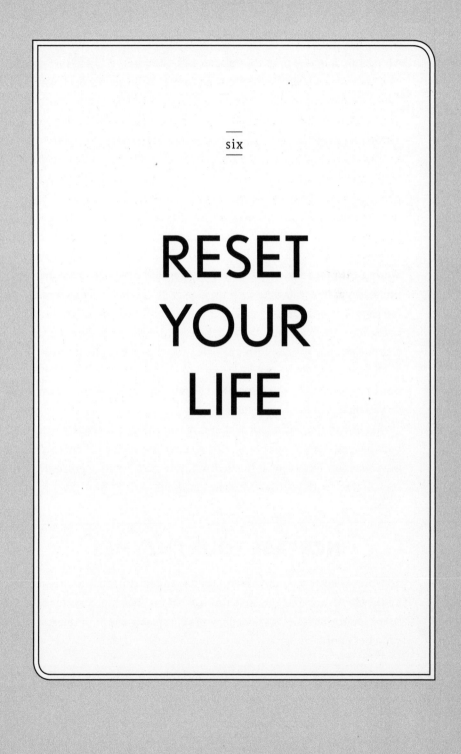

six

RESET YOUR LIFE

"You are never too old to set another goal or to dream a new dream."

—C. S. Lewis

During the Juice Cleanse Reset Diet, you bid farewell to toxins, unhealthy cravings, lackluster skin, bloat, and excess weight by feeding your body only healing and energizing foods. You not only eliminated the junk from your diet and the gunk from your body, but you also fueled your insides with antioxidants, enzymes, and vitamins. At this moment, you're in pristine fat-burning, toxin-flushing condition! You're officially reset. Now for the million-dollar question: how do you maintain long-term success?

Achieving long-term success and maintaining the postcleanse buzz happens choice by choice. This chapter is dedicated to increasing your knowledge and empowering you to make smart choices to stay on track with your reset for the long haul.

INCREASE YOUR ENZYMES

Enzymes are essential to vitality, beauty, and health; they are right up there with antioxidants in defining what makes many superfoods super. On the flip side, a lack of enzymes is arguably one of the biggest causes of poor health.

All bodily functions require enzymes. Enzymes are the catalysts for every activity, from the proper functioning of your internal organs, to your ability to think, to the detoxification and replenishment of your cells. If you still need more motivation for increasing your enzyme intake, how about this—a lack of enzymes is a guaranteed way to accelerate aging! Wrinkles, bone loss, weight gain, and even illness may all be attributed to enzyme deficiency. Without enzymes, outer beauty suffers because your cells cannot repair themselves. Even worse than this, if you consume both processed foods and real food, then the enzyme inhibitors in the processed foods can interfere with the enzymes from the real food you consume. This is one of the many reasons why we encourage you to stay away from processed food. As you age, your body produces fewer enzymes, requiring you to take in more from your food and supplements in order to avoid a deficiency.

There are three main types of enzymes: metabolic enzymes, digestive enzymes, and food enzymes. Metabolic enzymes are in charge of energy production in your body. Think of metabolic enzymes like your indispensable executive assistant for cellular activity on every level. These enzymes process the nutrients provided by your food and disperse them throughout your body to assist with replenishment of healthy cells. Metabolic enzymes also work overtime at no extra charge, helping you to flush toxins from your body. If you wish to give a little thank you for your metabolic enzymes, direct your gratitude toward your pancreas, the main organ that produces these hardworking overachievers and releases them into your body.

Digestive enzymes assist your body to break down and assimilate food into usable nutrients. Beginning with amylase in your saliva, enzymes go to work from the moment food hits your mouth. This is why it's important to chew your food before swallowing. It is also very beneficial to swish your juice and smoothies in your mouth for a moment before swallowing, because this will allow your digestive enzymes to get to work!

Your body requires different types of enzymes to digest fats, proteins, and carbohydrates.

Food enzymes primarily come from plants and are needed to break down food. Your body does not make these enzymes, but they are contained in the food you eat. Correction: they're contained in the food you eat if you eat real food that is not damaged by heat and processing. Because food enzymes are destroyed by heat, it's important to incorporate fresh raw fruits and vegetables into your daily diet as well as healthy essential cold-pressed or whole plant oils (for example, avocado or raw nuts) and, of course, juice or smoothies. Part of what made your juice-cleanse phase successful was the huge amount of enzymes that you consumed. Consuming enzymes through food boosts your body's ability to detox and repair without taxing your internal metabolic enzyme system. Feeding your body enzymes is how you lend a helping hand, eliminating a bit of the burden from your internal systems.

The excellent news is that throughout the Juice Cleanse Reset Diet, your body was flooded with enzymes and reset to crave more of them. This means you're already on the right path!

Now, take the money you're tempted to spend on creams, treatments, and injections, and put it toward the highest-quality, fresh, organic, raw fruits and vegetables and enzyme supplements that you can get your hands on. Dark green vegetables contain collagen-producing agents. Collagen is the main structural protein found in your connective tissue that keeps your skin firm, tight, and youthful. Eating kale, spinach, collards, and asparagus delivers key enzymes and nutrients that help strengthen your body's ability to manufacture and utilize collagen effectively. If you aren't consuming sufficient enzymes, you're left feeling hungry, lethargic, and undernourished, and your appearance is sure to reflect this situation. Increasing your enzyme intake will improve your beauty from the inside out.

Ways to Increase Your Enzymes

Fresh raw fruits and vegetables are the easiest place to get good food enzymes. Organics will deliver more than their conventional counterparts and will not come with a nasty side of pesticides.

Fermentation neutralizes enzyme inhibitors and breaks down gluten, sugars, and other difficult-to-digest elements of your food. Try our simple recipe for Fermented Veggies (page 189) or supplement your diet with Bragg Organic Apple Cider Vinegar, which may be purchased at most health food stores. Try a shot of it diluted in 4 ounces of water or mix it with organic olive oil as a salad dressing.

Much of the soil in which your food is grown contains significantly fewer minerals today than it did before modern farming and massive pollution took its toll. Mineral-depleted soil, yielding mineral-deficient crops, increases your risk for enzyme deficiency because one of the most important functions of minerals is to spark enzyme reactions within your body. For this reason, even many raw food followers supplement their diets with digestive enzymes (see page 108). Supplementation cannot make up for a diet that is void of all fruits, veggies, and fermented foods. However, enzyme supplements will alleviate some of the burden placed on your system by cooked food, depleted soil, and the few less-than-perfect meals you sneak in every once in a while. Taking enzymes after meals helps your body out a great deal. We highly recommend it!

SUPPLEMENT YOUR HEALTHY DIET

While you should aim to satisfy your nutrition needs mostly through your food, in today's busy world, it's not always possible. If you travel frequently, often eat meals away from home, or simply wish to increase your nutrient intake, smart supplementation may offer you a good solution.

Before you read the rest of this section, it's important for us to clarify that supplements cannot make up for a poor diet. Supplements are great for filling in the gaps and enhancing a healthy diet. If you're fulfilling your new healthy cravings post-reset, you're already including many more antioxidant-, vitamin-, and enzyme-rich foods in your diet than you were before you embarked on the Juice Cleanse Reset Diet.

The supplement suggestions we include in this section are the ones that our clients have most commonly needed and that have created significant changes in their digestive health, energy levels, and overall well-being. Please note that all of us have unique individual needs. You may only benefit from a few of the following suggestions or perhaps none. The recommended daily dosage and optimal time of consumption for each of these supplements is typically stated on the container and will vary based on the concentration and potency of each brand. We've given you a few of our preferred brands for each supplement we recommend. If you select a supplement that is outside of our suggestions, there are a few ingredients you should be careful to avoid.

- Hydrogenated oils: Chemically processed fat; used as a filler

- Artificial colors: Sometimes derived from toxic coal tar; used to make the vitamins look more appealing

- Titanium dioxide: Naturally occurring oxide of titanium. Can be contaminated with toxic lead; used as a pigment and to dilute potency

Remember to listen to your body and to check with your doctor before beginning any supplement program.

Probiotics

If you don't consume fermented foods at least a few times per week, have been on antibiotics for any length of time, or have suffered from digestive issues, you'll likely benefit from probiotic supplementation. Probiotics help your body assimilate food better, meaning that you'll retain more nutrients from all of the foods that you eat! Just as free radicals are everywhere and antioxidants are our defense mechanism, the ecology of our food system is such that bacteria are everywhere and probiotics are our first line of defense. Probiotics are especially beneficial for anyone who suffers from gut-damaging food sensitivities. After identifying and removing an offending food from your diet, the next step is to repair any damage that resulted from your history of consuming this food.

Good digestive health is critical to your overall health and happiness. Did you know that 75 percent of your immune system lives in your colon and small intestine? We have worked with countless clients who have suffered from chronic constipation for as long as they can remember, which causes discomfort and a host of other issues brought on by a sluggish bowel. Some of these clients, despite eating loads of fiber or even cycling on and off of laxatives, were still disappointed by the lack of action in the restroom. After adding a daily probiotic regimen, everything changed. Things began to move through and out with awesome regularity. Brands we love:

- Dr. Ohhira's Primal Defense contains twelve strains of friendly bacteria. Each capsule is fermented for three to five years for maximum potency and then individually wrapped to maintain freshness.

- Green Vibrance is a super addition to smoothies. Besides delivering twenty-five billion probiotics, it also provides nutrient-packed grasses like wheat grass and barley grass. We have seen the regular use of this single supplement greatly improve people's digestive health.

- Primal Defense by Garden of Life is a great option because it's a unique formula that contains a whole-food probiotic blend with Homeostatic Soil Organisms (HSOs). HSOs are the probiotics that you would get naturally if your food came from soil untouched by pesticides, herbicides, and other harmful chemicals.

Digestive Enzymes

The easier you can make your body's massive job of breaking down the food you eat, the more energy you'll have. Part of the reason the Juice Cleanse Reset Diet left you feeling energized was your insides were not working overtime to break down food. Living a processed food–free life puts you a giant leap ahead of where you were pre-reset. You can take even more of the burden off your digestive system's daily load by including digestive enzymes with your meals. Digestive enzymes come in extra handy for those meals that contain animal products like meat and dairy, which require extra work by your digestive system in order to break down properly. Brands we love:

- NCP (Natural Choice Products) Digestive Enzymes and Life-Give HHI-Zymes: Whether you use these or other brands, look for an option that delivers at least three kinds of enzymes. Your body needs protease, lipase, and cellulose, among others. Both of these brands offer you a full spectrum of digestive enzymes.

Protein Powder

When you're not cleansing, experiment with enhancing your smoothies with high-quality protein powder. This is a great way to increase your daily protein intake while giving your smoothie staying power. We suggest a plant protein (sprouted brown rice, hemp, or pea) or an organic, grass-fed, whey protein. A well-constructed smoothie—which includes a combination of greens for enzymes, fruit for fiber, and good-quality protein for amino acids—will keep you satisfied for four-plus hours. Brands we love:

- Epic Protein or Boku for plant-based proteins. Both of these start with USDA organic sprouted brown rice protein as the base and add an extra punch with superfoods.

- Protein 17 is free from fillers and sweeteners, making it the purest form of grass-fed whey protein on the market.

- Tera's Whey makes an organic whey protein that is readily available.

Vitamin D

It's been estimated that about one billion people around the globe suffer from vitamin D deficiency. Vitamin D production is stimulated by sun exposure. If you spend very little time outdoors, live in northern latitudes, or slather every inch of your body in sunscreen before stepping outside, it's possible you're deficient in vitamin D. The time you spend in your car does not count toward outdoor time because the sun does not stimulate vitamin D production when it's filtered through glass.

Unlike other vitamins, vitamin D is produced by your body in small quantities. Your body's ability to produce vitamin D makes it more like a hormone rather than a vitamin. Because your body self-regulates its vitamin D production, there's no chance of getting too much vitamin D from the sun! However, if your lifestyle lacks sufficient sun exposure, it is possible that you lack sufficient vitamin D. Moral of the story: get outside, and while you're out there, do something active. Twenty minutes of unprotected sun exposure is suggested for most people. With your beauty in mind, you can still protect your face, but leave some other parts exposed. Request a simple blood test from your doctor to see if your vitamin D levels are low. Brands we love:

- Metagenics, NOW, and Jarrow each make high-quality capsule forms of both vitamin D and vitamin D_3. Vitamin D is derived from plants. Vitamin D_3 is derived from animals. Although both supplements can satisfy your vitamin D needs, we suggest vitamin D_3 unless you're a vegan. Because it's not as easily absorbed, you may need to take vitamin D in higher dosages than you would take vitamin D_3.

Omega Fats

There are two types of essential—"essential" because your body does not produce them on its own—omega fats: omega-3 and omega-6. Both types are necessary for proper brain function, for healthy skin and hair, and for regulating your metabolism. Lately, omega-6s have been getting a bad rap because the standard American diet results in high levels of omega-6s and is often deficient in omega-3s. This off-balance ratio has been linked to various health problems, including heart disease. Unfortunately, this is not one of your body's self-regulating systems. You're responsible for striking the right balance between the two. The excellent news is that if you follow the Juice Cleanse Reset Diet, you're consuming a diet free from processed foods and this dramatically decreases your risk of consuming too many omega-6 fats. Instead, you can focus on ensuring that you are consuming enough omega-3s.

A Note on Beef

Grass-fed beef provides the correct ratio of omega-3s to omega-6s. However, when cows are fed corn and grain, they generate excessive amounts of omega-6, throwing off this ratio.

You can supplement with omega-3 from algae if you are a vegan. If you aren't, in addition to enjoying oily wild-caught fish weekly (think salmon and black cod), it's a good idea to take a high-quality omega-3 supplement that contains both EPA and DHA.

These powerful omegas have potent anti-inflammatory properties and contribute to heart health, joint health, increased brain function, and mood regulation. Choose a supplement brand that has been independently tested and is guaranteed to be free of heavy metals, such as mercury and lead, and other environmental toxins, including polychlorinated biphenyls, also known as PCBs. Brands we love:

- Carlson is one of our preferred brands. It's a high-quality omega-3 that contains EPA and DHA.

- Barlean's makes a product called Wild and Whole Krill Oil that we love. It's unfiltered, unrefined, and easily digestible.

CUT DOWN ON THE SUGAR

There are many different types of sugar and every nutrition expert has an opinion on which one is best. High-fructose corn syrup (HFCS) has taken the brunt of negativity in the war against sugar. While many experts argue that your body's biological response to HFCS may not be different than its response to any other sweetener, the chemically engineered sweetener represents the downside of processed foods in general. HFCS has made its way into about 80 percent of the processed foods that line the supermarket shelves, and most of it is genetically engineered. Good news: because you no longer consume processed foods, your intake of HFCS should be almost nonexistent.

In response to the consumer backlash against high-fructose corn syrup, soda companies are now beginning to change recipes and stamp their packaging with "Made with real sugar." Beware of emerging labels on food that are calling out their use of sugar as a

Sugar Substitutes to Avoid

Aspertame: An artificial sweetener that is 200 times sweeter than sugar. Avoid it! It's a sure marker of a highly processed food. While aspertame itself is calorie free, consumption of this fake sweetener is linked to increased hunger and overeating.

Maltitol, mannitol, and sorbitol: These are some of the common sugar alcohols found in plant matter. Despite often being positioned as healthy on food packaging, these sugar alcohols can cause grief for your digestion system and lead to weight gain.

good thing. Real sugar does not make soda a health food. Don't fall into this trap! Remember what we talked about in chapter 2: if a food label tells you how natural it is, chances are high that you're better off not eating it.

Regardless of its form, too much added sugar intake (meaning sugar that is not naturally occurring in the food) increases your risk of obesity, diabetes, elevated cholesterol, and high blood pressure. A 2010 study from Emory University and the U.S. Centers for Disease Control and Prevention showed that added sweeteners appear to raise triglycerides and lower HDL ("good") cholesterol levels. Here is a brief explanation of some of the nonsugar options available. Whichever you decide to make your go-to source, use it in moderation!

- Agave: Extracted from the core of the agave plant. Agave is 1.4 to 1.6 times sweeter tasting than sugar, which allows you to use less of it to achieve the same sweetness as sugar. Rich in trace minerals.

- Coconut sugar: Produced from the sap of cut flower buds of the coconut palm. Its subtle sweetness and lower glycemic index make it one of our favorite sweeteners. Similar to brown sugar in taste but with a far superior nutrient profile, coconut sugar is an option to try as an alternative to regular sugar.

- Honey: Naturally antimicrobial and antibacterial. Many people report that adding a small amount of raw honey from your local area can bolster your resistance to environmental allergens.

- Maple syrup: Both grade A (light in color) and grade B (dark in color) maple syrup have trace minerals, but choose the darker grade B option for more calcium.

MOVE EVERY DAY

There are many reasons that you need to move daily. Proper detoxification is one of the most important of these reasons. Your lymph system carries nutrients to your cells and transports waste products away. In contrast to your blood, which is automatically pumped by the heart, your lymph system depends on physical activity in order to function properly. Without adequate physical activity, your cells are left swimming in their own waste products and starving for nutrients. This is one of the many things that can contribute to toxin overload.

Were you successful at changing your eating in the past, but have never formed a steady workout program? Or have you been disciplined with workouts only to go and ruin your workout with an unhealthy meal or eating too much? Now is the time to pull all of the pieces together for long-lasting benefits and results! Frequent and consistent exercise (regardless of the form) is a key component of the Reset Your Life plan.

Exercise Resets

Adding exercise to your life will deliver unparalleled immediate and long-term results that you'll feel and see. It's a surefire way to sustain the results you have already achieved and to continue to improve your health. Exercise supports all seven categories of resets.

Reset Your Attitude and Your Mindset

Exercise triggers the release of endorphins, increasing your serotonin levels and boosting your happiness. Attitude is everything.

Reset Your Energy

Frequent exercise revs up your energy levels by strengthening your cardiovascular system, allowing you to move through life with ease and energy!

Reset Your Metabolism

Exercise purifies your blood and carries fresh oxygen to your cells, increasing metabolism and fat assimilation.

Reset Your Taste Buds

Adding exercise to your day leaves you feeling empowered and makes it less likely that you will crave junk food. When you feel good, choosing healthy food is much easier.

Reset Your Digestive System

Exercise invigorates your lymphatic system, prompting the elimination of waste products and freeing up your liver to focus on burning fat.

Reset Your Weight

Exercise is proven to be the best way to combat stress, which results in fat retention. The stress-busting and calorie-burning effects of exercise make it an essential component for maintaining your optimal weight.

Reset Your Beauty

Sweat purges your body of toxins that can clog your pores and plague you with dull and lackluster skin.

While it may not be in the form of traditional exercise, we aim to be active every day and to walk at least 10,000 steps even on days we don't go to the gym. You should aim to do the same. Get yourself a pedometer (they can be purchased for as little as $10) and aim for 10,000 steps per day. If you never go the gym and never commit to a formal workout but can fit 10,000 steps per day into your life, your fitness will be elevated and maintaining your reset will be much easier.

JAMES T., INVESTMENT BANKER • For many years, I have worked really long hours, borderline workaholic status. When I bundled that with having a wife plus two awesome kids who are involved in multiple sports, I felt a giant amount of guilt any time I chose to work out. I wanted the little free time I had to be spent with my family.

I knew my health needed some serious attention because I was constantly tired and felt generally unenthusiastic about life, but I wanted a solution that would not take up any more of my time. The Juice Cleanse Reset Diet seemed to be the perfect solution. I was willing to commit seven days to getting my health on track, and my wife felt the recipes were something she could make for herself and our children as well.

My results were dramatic. I lost eight pounds in three days and I felt great. Upon completing that cleanse, I embarked on the Reset Your Life, and worked with Lori and Marra to see how I could really tailor it to my lifestyle. Besides the changes in my eating, they asked me to commit to taking any business phone calls after the stock market closed for the day on my cell phone instead of at my desk. This allows me to take some of my afternoon calls as I walk around the block or through the office rather than tying me to my desk. I use a pedometer and just by walking and talking I reach almost 8,000 steps per day. I lost another two pant sizes in just two months and my energy is back to where it used to be! My children eat the same meals I do, and wouldn't even think of asking for chicken fingers for dinner anymore. They even love the green juices and ask my wife to make them a juice or smoothie when they come home from practice each day.

Know your personality and then figure out a way to fit in more activity. If walking to the store is not realistic for you, pledge to park in the furthest parking spot. If you live in a temperate climate, make an effort to get outside more. Consider meeting a friend for an activity or to go for a walk instead of meeting for cocktails or coffee. As long as you're able-bodied, some form of daily activity must be a part of your wellness plan. Choose what you enjoy, whether it be Pilates, yoga, classes at your local gym, walking, running, or hiking.

What will it take for you to commit to moving more? Do you need a workout buddy for accountability? Do you need to schedule an allotted time for exercise into your calendar? Do you need to invest in a trainer, gym membership, proper apparel, or some simple home equipment? Or do you just need a pedometer to start tracking your steps? The exercise that is right for you won't necessarily be the same that is right for your neighbor, sister, spouse, or best friend. Find something that makes sense for you and your lifestyle. We're sure you've heard it before, but the best exercise is the kind that you'll do!

MINDY J., EXECUTIVE ASSISTANT • With a full-time job and three kids, working out for long stretches of time isn't feasible for me right now. I first completed the Juice Cleanse Reset Diet a year ago with good results. Because I had reset my taste buds and I was making better food choices, I continued to lose weight after completing my initial seven-day cleanse. However, eventually I plateaued before reaching my final goal weight. Because my schedule wasn't conducive to long workout sessions, Lori and Marra suggested that I invest in a mini trampoline and work up to two fifteen-minute jumping sessions per day. I followed their recommendation and the results have been remarkable. I didn't think I could feel better than I had post-reset, but adding in this bit of exercise helped my energy soar to a whole new level. Plus my elimination improved, and best of all, I beat that stubborn plateau.

PREPARE REAL FOOD AT HOME

Now that you have made the commitment to eat better, you'll need to make a commitment to putting more time into preparing what you're going to eat. Meals made from scratch will be more nutritious, more delicious, and less expensive than meals taken out of a box and thrown in the microwave. But they are also more time intensive to prepare.

To set yourself up for success, choose one day to cook for the entire week. That way, you won't be tempted to cheat just because you're short on time. By making a habit of taking a couple of hours to cook on the weekend, you'll save time during the week. You won't have to worry about what to eat each evening, or whether you need to run to the store. You'll have all the ingredients on hand.

Below you'll find a shopping list, menu, and recipes for everything you need for one week. You can adjust the menu to include any of the recipes in chapter 8. Stick to drinking a smoothie or juice every morning, pack up your lunch and snack, and revel in the ease of enjoying a home-cooked meal every weeknight with only minutes of preparation. Although we haven't specifically listed it below, you need to continue drinking 16 ounces of water at every meal and at least 8 ounces with each snack.

Shopping List for Menu Planning

We created a shopping list (see pages 118–120) for the weeklong menu plan that follows. If you're a vegetarian, shopping and preparing will be easier for you: simply stock up on unprocessed, canned beans and nuts, including black beans, garbanzo beans, cooked lentils, and so on. Any time a recipe calls for an animal product, either add more veggies, some nuts, or a cup of beans in place of the protein. You can also use quinoa in place of the animal protein.

SHOPPING LIST

- ☐ 1 (5- to 6-pound) whole organic roasting chicken
- ☐ 2 pounds organic ground turkey
- ☐ 4 boneless, skinless organic chicken breasts
- ☐ 1 pound large shrimp, peeled and deveined
- ☐ 1½ pounds jumbo sea scallops
- ☐ 12 ounces firm white fish, such as halibut or cod
- ☐ 1 (14.5-ounce) can organic, low-sodium vegetable broth
- ☐ 1 (14.5-ounce) can tomato sauce
- ☐ 1 (14.5-ounce) can diced tomatoes
- ☐ 1 (8-ounce) can tomato paste
- ☐ 1 (14.5-ounce) can organic black beans
- ☐ 1 (14.5-ounce) can organic garbanzo beans
- ☐ 1 pound quinoa
- ☐ 1 pound brown rice
- ☐ 1 head butter lettuce
- ☐ 1 head each red leaf and green leaf romaine, or 2 (1-pound) bags mixed baby greens
- ☐ 3 pounds loose baby spinach, or 3 (1-pound) bags baby spinach
- ☐ 3 bunches loose kale, or 3 (6-ounce) bags chopped kale
- ☐ 1 head garlic
- ☐ 1 (1-inch) piece fresh ginger
- ☐ 4 heads baby bok choy
- ☐ 4 medium cucumbers

- ❏ 4 carrots
- ❏ 2 (8-ounce) bags shredded organic carrots, or 2 pounds loose carrots, shredded
- ❏ 1 (8-ounce) bag baby carrots
- ❏ 1 pineapple
- ❏ 4 green bell peppers
- ❏ 6 red bell peppers
- ❏ 2 orange or yellow bell peppers
- ❏ 4 medium zucchini
- ❏ 3 large summer squash
- ❏ 2 heads broccoli, or 2 (8-ounce) bags broccoli florets
- ❏ 1 pint cherry tomatoes
- ❏ 3 (16-ounce) containers organic strawberries, or 3 (16-ounce) bags frozen organic strawberries
- ❏ 2 (4-ounce) containers organic fresh blueberries, or 1 (8-ounce) bag frozen organic blueberries
- ❏ 2 (4-ounce) containers organic fresh raspberries, or 1 (8-ounce) bag frozen raspberries
- ❏ 5 bananas
- ❏ 8 Granny Smith apples
- ❏ 1 red apple (any variety)
- ❏ 4 pears
- ❏ 2 avocados
- ❏ 2 white onions
- ❏ 1 spaghetti squash
- ❏ 4 lemons

SHOPPING LIST, continued

- ❑ 8 ounces raw walnuts
- ❑ 14 ounces raw cashews
- ❑ 2 pounds raw almonds
- ❑ 8 ounces dried cranberries
- ❑ 8 ounces cacao nibs
- ❑ 8 ounces chia seeds
- ❑ 1 small loaf whole-grain bread
- ❑ 1 (16-ounce) container steel-cut oats
- ❑ Salt-free seasoning, such as lemon pepper, 21 Seasoning Salute, or other
- ❑ 1 (8-ounce) container organic hummus (or another can of garbanzo beans to make your own)
- ❑ 1 (8-ounce) container Greek yogurt
- ❑ 1 (4-ounce) container pico de gallo
- ❑ 1 (8-ounce) bottle olive oil
- ❑ 1 (8-ounce) bottle Bragg Liquid Aminos
- ❑ 1 (8-ounce) bottle organic coconut water
- ❑ 1 dozen large eggs
- ❑ 4 ounces shredded low-fat cheddar cheese (optional)
- ❑ 4 ounces shredded parmesan cheese
- ❑ 8 ounces crumbled low-fat feta cheese (optional)

Preparation Day

If you set aside a few hours one day, you can prepare your proteins and other time-consuming foods for the entire week. You'll pack your lunches more quickly in the morning, and you won't make excuses at dinnertime. If you can whip up a healthy meal for your family in twenty minutes, there is no reason to grab takeout, even on the busiest days.

1. Roast the whole chicken and chicken breasts according to the recipes on page 194 and 196. Once cooled, cut the breasts into slices and shred the dark meat from the thighs and legs of the roasted chicken. Store in an airtight container in the refrigerator.

2. Season the ground turkey with the salt-free seasoning. In a large sauté pan over medium heat, cook the turkey in two batches, tossing constantly until the meat is no longer pink. Store covered in the refrigerator for up to 5 days.

3. Roast the peppers, zucchini, squash, and broccoli in the oven according to the recipe for a double batch of Roasted Garden Vegetables (page 209). Store covered in the refrigerator for up to 5 days.

4. Prepare 2 cups of the quinoa according to the Cooked Quinoa recipe (page 206). Store covered in the refrigerator for up to 7 days.

5. Prepare 2 cups of brown rice according to Brown Rice recipe (page 207). Store covered in the refrigerator for up to 7 days.

6. Soak the almonds and make a double batch of homemade Almond Milk (page 181). Store in sealed 16-ounce glass mason jars in the refrigerator for up to 4 days.

7. Make a double batch of Ritual Trail Mix (page 194). Separate into ½-cup portions and store in resealable plastic bags in a cool, dark place.

Now you're ready for the week. If you follow the meal plan below, you'll be on your way to resetting for life.

MEAL PLAN

This plan consists of three meals and one snack per day. If you weigh over 175 pounds, you should add another smoothie, juice, or snack to each day. You may choose any from the juice, smoothie, or snack recipes in chapter 8.

Day 1

Breakfast
16 ounces water
Green Berry Smoothie (page 174)

Lunch
16 ounces water
Mediterranean Salad (page 186)
If you're taking it with you to work, store the salad in a container without the dressing and bring 2 ounces of the dressing in another container. When you're ready for lunch, add the dressing to the salad, cover, shake, and enjoy.

Snack
16 ounces water
Handful raw almonds
1 small apple

Dinner
16 ounces water
Mixed Green Salad (page 188) with Lemon Vinaigrette (page 212)
One breast and one leg from your Roast Chicken (page 194), skin removed
1 cup Roasted Garden Vegetables (page 209)
½ cup Cooked Quinoa (page 206), reheated or served cold

Day 2

Breakfast

16 ounces water

Green Almond Smoothie (page 173)

Lunch

16 ounces water

1 (8-ounce) scoop Chicken Salad (page 190) on mixed greens
with your choice of vinaigrette (page 211) or 1 slice toasted
whole-wheat bread, or 1 cup Roasted Garden Vegetables (page
209) on mixed greens with your choice of vinaigrette (page 211)

Snack

16 ounces water

16 baby carrots with 2 tablespoons Hummus (page 191)

Dinner

16 ounces water

3 large scallops, sautéed

Sautéed Spinach (page 211)

½ cup cooked Brown Rice (page 207)

Tomato-Avocado Salad (page 184)

Day 3

Breakfast

16 ounces water

Green Banana Smoothie (page 173)

Lunch

16 ounces water

Roasted Veggie and Chicken Salad (page 186)

If you're taking it with you to work, store the salad in a container without the dressing and bring 2 ounces of the dressing
in another container. When you're ready for lunch, add the
dressing to the salad, cover, shake, and enjoy.

Snack

16 ounces water

½ cup Greek yogurt with ½ cup blueberries

Dinner
16 ounces water
Shrimp Stir-Fry (page 201, variation)

Day 4

Breakfast
16 ounces water
Pineapple-Banana Smoothie (page 178)

Lunch
16 ounces water
Spinach Salad (page 185)
6 ounces Roasted Chicken Breast (page 196)
2 tablespoons Balsamic Vinaigrette (page 212)

Snack
16 ounces water
1 cup Chia Seed Pudding (page 193)

Dinner
16 ounces water
Small Mixed Green Salad (page 188) with vinaigrette of choice
   (see page 211)
Turkey-Stuffed Peppers (page 209)

Day 5

Breakfast
16 ounces water
Green Almond Smoothie (page 173)

Lunch
16 ounces water
Kale-Quinoa Salad (page 187)

Snack
16 ounces water
½ cup Ritual Trail Mix (page 194)

Dinner
16 ounces water
Butter Lettuce Tacos (page 195)

Day 6

Breakfast
16 ounces water
Roasted Vegetable Frittata (page 183)

Lunch
16 ounces water
Mediterranean Salad (page 186)
Raw Red Pepper Soup (page 206)

Snack
16 ounces water
1 cup Greek yogurt with ½ cup blueberries

Dinner
16 ounces water
Spaghetti Squash with Turkey Marinara Sauce (page 202)

Day 7

Breakfast
16 ounces water
Strawberry-Banana Smoothie (page 176)

Lunch
16 ounces water
Roasted Vegetable Frittata (page 183)
Mixed Green Salad (page 188) with vinaigrette of choice
    (page 211)

Snack
16 ounces water
1 cup Chia Seed Pudding (page 204)

Dinner
16 ounces water
Fish Baked in Foil (page 198)
Kale-Quinoa Salad (page 187)

This meal plan was created to give you the opportunity to try out some of our recipes, but we want you to enjoy the flexibility and freedom of choosing other meals or smoothies or snacks from the plan in order to find your own favorites. The main point is to learn to plan ahead for lifetime success.

Although we have included a full meal plan for all seven days, we understand that you may have a cheat meal each week. Some of you may love Sunday brunch, others may look forward to their Saturday night "date night" and wish to have freedom there. We generally reserve our splurges for social activities, knowing there are bound to be one or two each week, and stick to healthy, nutritious, sound whole food meals in between. Listen to your body, recognize the impact of your lifestyle on your choices, and tweak the plan to work for you.

TAILOR THESE PRINCIPLES TO YOUR LIFESTYLE

We have covered a lot of different topics in this chapter, including how and why you should increase your enzymes, how to supplement your diet, what the differences are among sugar options, and why it's so important to find an exercise program that you can stick with. We've even given you a full week's worth of recipes to show you how easy it is to integrate this new way of eating into your life.

All of this new information may seem a little overwhelming, but the main questions for you to consider are these: What can you commit to every day? What healthy habits can you add in each week?

The key to your long-term success lies in making small changes that you feel most comfortable with and that best fit into your life. You may opt to eat more salads, choose organic whenever possible, stay away from processed foods on a daily basis—all of these are great starting points. Celebrate your successes and brush off the slipups. Remember that what you do the majority of the time has the most impact on your results. At times when you seek greater and more noticeable results, you now know how to intensify your game. You can always revert back to the Juice Cleanse Reset Diet protocol, and if you have a special occasion coming up and you want to make big changes quickly, check out our supercharged cleanses in chapter 7.

The main message we want to communicate to you in regard to tailoring the program to your life is to choose your priorities. You can't do everything all of the time. Create a list of the things you can commit to, and then prioritize your list in order to keep your reset going.

Our priority list looks like this:

- Drink lots of filtered water every day
- Buy 100 percent organic for at-home meals
- Start each morning with a juice or smoothie
- Take probiotics
- Prepare dinner at home at least three days per week
- Exercise at least four days per week

During times when you need to clean up your diet, make sure you schedule all of your diet priorities onto your calendar so that they happen. Other times, schedule as much as you can. Celebrate with a mental pat on the back when you accomplish everything that is scheduled. Commit to getting over it quickly when you don't get to everything on your list. Focus on moving forward in the right direction rather than harping on the past.

Before we close this chapter, let's take a moment to reflect on all you have accomplished. You've cleaned out the toxins, flooded your body with nutrients, learned how to exercise and eat right, and you have delicious, nutritious, inexpensive recipes you can use over and over again. You've probably lost a few pounds, and have seen noticeable changes in your skin and appearance. You're armed with a newly reset attitude, energy level, and metabolism. Your body craves healthy nutritious food, your digestive system works much more efficiently, and you are radiant!

Although you're prepared to make the best decisions in the future, there'll be those times when you gain a few pounds, or get off track, or just find yourself in a rut. Don't get down on yourself; just get back to real, whole foods. In the next chapter, we have three different plans to help you get back on track when you need a serious reset in a hurry or in a more significant way. You can save these plans for those little emergencies, or you can use them if you feel you still have more work to do and want to continue losing weight, repairing your beauty, or getting toned. Read on to supercharge!

seven

SUPER-CHARGED RESETS FOR MOMENTOUS OCCASIONS

"Patience and perseverance have a magical effect before which difficulties disappear and obstacles vanish."

—John Quincy Adams

We've all been there: you had the best intentions of getting in shape for a momentous occasion months in advance, but somehow your health, the craziness of work, the demands of your family, unexpected travels, or pure procrastination derailed those intentions. Suddenly your big event is weeks or even days away, and you need a plan to help you look and feel amazing ASAP. It happens. We get it. In fact, the supercharged resets provided in this chapter were designed especially for these situations.

Everyone from celebrities getting ready for the red carpet to couples preparing for their wedding day have used these supercharged resets to get visible results quickly. The more closely you live the Reset Your Life principles, the less necessary the supercharged resets become. Still, we believe 100 percent in using momentous occasions as your catalyst for stepping up your game and making bigger changes in your self-care and your diet.

If you're motivated to present your best self at your upcoming event, following one of the supercharged reset programs from this chapter is definitely in order! Knowing you'll be showing all in a swimsuit on that tropical vacation or needing to fit into a slim pair of suit pants or a slinky black dress for that class reunion is a surefire way to make you kick your wellness rituals into high gear. Capitalize on how motivated you feel at this moment and dive in with total dedication. Determine your personal goal for the event and then choose the category below that best fits your needs and time frame:

Supercharged Reset #1: Reset Your Weight in 21 Days
Press the reset button, drop ten pounds, restore your glow (page 144).

Supercharged Reset #2: Reset Your Health in 10 Days
Lose five pounds, tighten up, eliminate cravings (page 156).

Supercharged Reset #3: Reset and Refresh in 3 Days
Banish bloat, get refreshed, be confident (page 160).

Consider the supercharged resets to be your crash course in overall wellness. Just as in the Juice Cleanse Reset Diet, your success will require some advance planning and your complete dedication.

The supercharged resets cover the standard seven main areas—your attitude and your mindset, your energy, your metabolism, your taste buds, your digestive system, your weight, and your beauty—as well as an eighth: exercise. Because these supercharged resets are designed to achieve significant and visible results, they emphasize beauty and exercise. Therefore, to help guarantee that you'll meet your desired goal, we go into more detail on how to reset your beauty and your exercise. Exercise plays an important part in the twenty-one- and ten-day supercharged resets because it can enhance the results of all of the other resets! If you've been unsuccessful at sticking to a consistent exercise routine, now is the time for you to change that. Follow the program we give you, and you'll be amazed by the results.

THE SUPERCHARGED RESETS

Reset Your Attitude and Your Mindset

Keep your eye on the prize. Supercharged resets are the absolutely perfect time to focus your attention on a tangible goal. Visualize with perfect detail fitting into the dress or slacks that you want to wear for your special occasion. Focus on this goal throughout your super-charged reset and you'll maintain the motivation you need in order to stay on course.

Reset Your Energy

Fueling your body with nature's best fruits and vegetables, having a goal that motivates you, and bringing more mindfulness into your days will help your energy skyrocket. Use the supercharged resets as an opportunity to free yourself from the burden of life-force depleting foods and toxic thoughts.

Reset Your Metabolism

The combination of replacing processed foods with natural, pure foods and increasing the frequency with which you feed your cells good nutrition can improve your metabolism and bring your body back to functioning at its optimal level.

Reset Your Taste Buds

If you have veered off track since your initial experience with the Juice Cleanse Reset Diet, it's time to get back to basics when it comes to good nutrition. Say good-bye to added sugars, refined carbohy-drates, and chemically engineered foods. The supercharged resets lead you back to real foods and, ultimately, leave you with cravings for unprocessed, nutrient-rich fresh food.

Reset Your Digestive System

The important addition of oxygen-carrying, organ-cleansing, and enzyme-rich leafy greens to your diet helps restore good digestion. Supercharged resets can wake up sluggish bowels and improve overall digestion.

Reset Your Weight

Consider the supercharged resets to be your ultimate jump start toward skinny. The combination of what you're eating, what you're eliminating, detox treatments, and exercise will help you shed pounds and shrink your waistline.

RESET YOUR BEAUTY

Not only do the foods in the supercharged resets make you glow from the inside out, but the facial and body treatments we include in this section also help you glow on the outside. Use these simple and effective ways to restore a more youthful glow in time for your special occasion.

Supercharged resets are the perfect time to pamper yourself. Make the time to squeeze in facial and body treatments on the specified days. These treatments are designed to enhance your beauty and to open up your pores to allow for the elimination of toxins through your skin.

Facials, Brighteners, and Lighteners

Indulge in the natural and effective facial and body recipes below to improve the appearance and texture of your skin. Even if you have sensitive skin and have found that store-bought facial treatments are too harsh, you may find the natural and gentle recipes below to be a perfect fit. You'll be amazed at how easy to prepare and beneficial these at-home recipes are for your skin.

Pineapple and Coconut Milk Hydrating Facial

Perfect for restoring hydration and remedying dry or flaky skin. Pineapple is amazing for reducing inflammation and puffiness. Coconut milk provides nourishing and easily absorbed hydration. Watch redness and puffiness disappear, leaving glowing skin.

4 slices fresh pineapple
2 tablespoons coconut milk

Combine the pineapple and coconut milk in a food processor and puree until smooth. Spread the paste uniformly over your face and leave on for 10 minutes. Remove with a damp cloth.

Greek Yogurt and Lemon Facial Skin Tightener

This gently exfoliating treatment gives you lifted and firm-looking skin instantly. Lemons slough away dead skin and Greek yogurt's antibacterial properties prevent skin breakouts. Lactic acid in the yogurt shrinks pores, leaving you with more youthful-looking skin. This skin tightener can be done two or three times a week or whenever your skin needs a lift.

2 tablespoons plain Greek yogurt
Juice of 1 lemon
1 tablespoon honey

In a small bowl, combine the yogurt, lemon juice, and honey and stir until smooth. Apply to your cleansed face and neck. Allow it to dry for 20 to 30 minutes. Leave it on until you feel the skin tighten or up to 1 hour. When ready, rinse with tepid water followed by a cold rinse.

Pulp and Honey Skin Brightener

After making any juice with carrots, beets, or sweet potato in it, use the leftover pulp as the base for an antioxidant-rich mask. This will give you an immediately refreshed and glowing look. Honey helps hold moisture in the skin. It has astringent properties to draw out impurities that would normally stay clogged and cause blemishes. This mask is non-drying and your face should feel nice and smooth afterward. Orange- and red-pigmented produce have natural antiseptic properties with skin-brightening effects.

1/2 cup carrot pulp (or other red- or orange-pigmented pulp, such as sweet potato and beet)
1 tablespoon raw honey

In a small bowl, combine the carrot pulp and honey until a paste forms. Apply to your clean skin. Allow it to stay on for 10 to 15 minutes and rinse with warm water. Pat dry.

Yogurt Base Skin Lightener

This mask will quickly become your new secret weapon for dealing with freckles, sunspots, or overall discoloration. Turmeric is fantastic for evening out skin discolorations. Lemons slough away dead skin.

3 or 4 almonds, or 1 tablespoon almond meal
1 1/2 cups plain organic yogurt
2 tablespoons freshly squeezed lemon juice
1 teaspoon honey
Pinch of ground turmeric

Use a food processor to crush the almonds into powder. Combine the almonds with the remaining ingredients and stir vigorously to blend well. Apply a small amount of the lightener to your skin. Leave it on for 1 to 2 hours before rinsing your face.

Mint and Lavender Facial

This refreshing and skin-soothing facial is multifunctional. Lavender and mint help induce relaxation, awaken your senses, and promote clear thinking, while the eggs help tighten and tone your skin.

1 teaspoon organic raw honey
1 raw egg
1 teaspoon dried lavender
1 teaspoon fresh chopped mint

Warm the honey in a small pan over low heat and then blend with the egg to form a creamy paste. Add the lavender and mint and stir into the paste. Cover your face and neck with this soothing facial and leave it on for 15 minutes, or until it dries. Remove the mask with a damp cloth to reveal a more relaxed you.

GEORGIA T., PEDIATRIC NURSE • The carrot and honey facial mask has completely changed my skin. Store-bought skin treatments are too harsh for me. The brightening result this simple mixture creates is amazing!

Body Treatments

If you haven't ever experienced an at-home body treatment, you're in for a treat. Not only will these treatments flush toxins from your skin, but they'll also leave your skin radiant and smooth.

Coffee Ground Exfoliant

Caffeic acid, found in coffee, has great anti-inflammatory and anti-oxidant effects on the skin. It improves skin elasticity by stimulating collagen production. This one is a bit messy, but the silky and smooth results are definitely worth a little mess.

> 1 cup warm coffee grounds
> $^1\!/_2$ cup sea salt
> 2 tablespoons olive oil

Lay newspapers down on your bathroom floor. Stir all ingredients together and apply the mixture to dry skin. Brush thoroughly onto skin, giving extra attention to your elbows, feet, and other extra dry areas. Leave on for about 2 minutes. Brush off as much of the mixture as possible before hopping in the shower. Alternatively, you can apply and wash off in the shower, but cover the drain with mesh to avoid clogging.

Banana-Sugar Scrub

We have to share this one because it's one of the best uses for brown bananas (in addition to freezing them for smoothies). Bananas that have started to brown have higher potassium levels than yellow bananas, which is partially why this scrub results in such beautiful and well-hydrated skin. The sugar sloughs away the dead skin cells, allowing your skin to soak in the potassium.

> 1 ripe banana
> 3 tablespoons granulated sugar
> $^1\!/_4$ teaspoon pure vanilla extract or your favorite essential oil
> (optional)

Smash ingredients together with a fork into a chunky consistency. In the shower, pat the sugar mixture over your body and gently massage it in. Rinse off with warm water. Bonus: break off a small piece of the banana peel and rub the inside part of it on your teeth for about 60 seconds for whiter teeth. Some call this an old wives' tale, but it works for us! Try it for yourself before throwing away the peel.

Easy DIY Body Scrub

If you're juicing, combine the leftover pulp from any juice you make with Himalayan sea salt for an effective body scrub.

RESET YOUR EXERCISE

Fat-burning aerobic exercise (*aerobic* means "with oxygen") is an important component of the supercharged resets because it allows you to maintain muscle mass, decrease unsightly cellulite, and rid your body of stored toxins that have made themselves at home in your fat cells. Fat-burning exercise, achieved by keeping your heart rate below a certain threshold (we explain how to determine this threshold below), burns the maximum percentage of calories from fat, revs up your metabolism, and promotes serious sweating. An example of fat-burning aerobic exercise is simply walking at a moderate pace.

In addition to your normal strength-training program (if you have one), you'll do this low-intensity, fat-burning cardio session on an empty stomach upon rising each day. Your glycogen levels (stored carbohydrates) are lowest after fasting for eight hours while sleeping. For this reason, a morning workout that is completed upon rising allows for maximum fat burning.

For the fat-burning and toxin-flushing tasks at hand, your morning exercise is one of the times in life when less intensity yields better results. Because your overall calorie consumption will be lower than normal during the supercharged reset, your goal is to exercise while avoiding burnout and excessive hunger. Avoid making the mistake of working out at full effort in hopes of burning massive calories. The intention for your morning workout is not to burn the maximum amount of calories, but rather to burn the highest percentage of calories from fat as possible in order to get your lymphatic system moving. This maximizes fat loss and reduces your toxic load.

Let Your Liver Burn Fat

High-energy activity that leaves you breathless can build up lactic acid. While lactic acid is a completely normal by-product of anaerobic (*anaerobic* means "absence of oxygen") respiration, this acid is converted into pyruvate by your liver, which allows you to continue pushing through an intense portion of your workout despite the lack of available oxygen. Part of the beauty of staying within the low-intensity, fat-burning, aerobic zone during your morning workout is that instead of dealing with the conversion of lactic acid into pyruvate, your liver can stay focused on metabolizing fat for elimination.

Find Your Ideal Training Zones

Because exercising within your fat-burning zone is an important part of the reset, you may want to consider investing in a heart rate monitor. Good-quality heart rate monitors start around $30.

To identify your ideal training zone using a heart rate monitor:

1. First determine your resting heart rate (RHR). While sitting still before doing any exercise, see how many times per minute your heart beats. Record that number.

2. Once you know your RHR, determine your ideal fat-burning zone using the Karvonen formula: to determine the lower range, you figure 220 minus [your age] minus [your RHR] x 60% + [your RHR]. To determine the upper range, you figure 220 minus [your age] minus [your RHR] x 70% + [your RHR]. See the sidebar below for an example.

Determine Your Target Heart Rate

If you're 40 years old with a resting heart rate of 65 and you want to know your training heart rate for the intensity level of 60 to 70 percent:

Lower range: 220 - 40 [age] = 180, 180 - 65 [RHR] = 115, 115 x .60 [minimum intensity] + 65[RHR]=134 beats/minute.

Upper range: 220 - 40 [age] = 180, 180 - 65 [RHR] = 115, 115 x .70 [maximum intensity] + 65 [RHR] = 146 beats/minute.

Training at the 60 to 70 percent intensity level means your training heart rate zone should be 134 to 146 beats per minute.

To find your ideal training zone without using a heart rate monitor: If you don't own a heart rate monitor and it's not on your list of priority purchases, use this rate of perceived exertion (RPE) section in order to evaluate your workout intensity. You should aim to stay within zone 2 for the most efficient fat-torching results.

Zone 1: Easy-breezy/50 to 60 percent of maximum effort or percentage of maximum heart rate:

- You could do it all day if it weren't for boredom or blisters. This zone is often used as a warm-up for activity. Consistently exercising in this zone has been shown to decrease body fat, blood pressure, and cholesterol.
- Up to 85 percent of calories burned are from fat.

Zone 2: Easy fat burning/about 60 to 70 percent of maximum effort or percentage of maximum heart rate:

- You can carry on a conversation with ease.
- You experience the same benefits as zone 1, but more total calories are burned.
- Up to 85 percent of calories burned are from fat.

Zone 3: Moderate aerobic/about 70 to 80 percent of maximum effort or percentage of maximum heart rate:

- You can speak but need to catch your breath after a few sentences.
- Exercise at this level improves cardiovascular and respiratory systems and strengthens your heart.
- More calories are burned, but the percentage of fat burned drops down to about 50 percent.

Zone 4: Challenging anaerobic/about 80 to 90 percent of maximum effort or percentage of maximum heart rate:

- You definitely can't speak with any ease.
- You could sustain this pace for two minutes.
- This is the zone where you improve your VO_2 max (the amount of oxygen you consume during exertion) and endurance.

- In this high-intensity zone, you burn maximum calories but only about 15 percent from fat.

Zone 5: Maximum exertion/about 90 to 100 percent of maximum effort or percentage of maximum heart rate:

- The zone is only sustainable for very short durations (sixty seconds max).
- You must catch your breath after a short time at this level.

Now that you understand where your target heart rate or your perceived rate of exertion should be, you're ready to add fat-flushing cardio into your life. In order to guarantee maximum results, the supercharged resets give you the exact duration of time you should be in your zone each day. Make it happen!

ALLISON C., STAY-AT-HOME MOM • I followed the twenty-one day supercharged reset before going to Hawaii for my ten-year anniversary with my hubby. After having three babies in the last six years, I had major anxiety about being out in daylight in my bikini. The anxiety was more about how I would feel than it was about what my husband would see. I spoke with Lori and Marra about doing a supercharged reset and I decided to dive in. Of course, the shift in my food intake made a difference, but I truly believe that the fat-burning morning cardio is what created the biggest difference in my waistline. Each morning I would sweat completely through my clothing and it felt like the fat was just melting away! Fast-forward to Hawaii and, I am thrilled to say, I felt confident and beautiful in my swimsuit.

Integrate Strength Training into Your Workout

We are big advocates of strength training for longevity, overall health, and long-term weight-loss success. Still, strength training is an optional component of your supercharged resets. For aesthetic purposes, we emphasize fat-burning workouts over strength training during supercharged resets. If you have beautiful muscles but they are hidden below a layer of fat, you'll still feel underwhelmed with your appearance on your big day.

If you already have a strength-training routine, feel free to continue. This could be Pilates, weight lifting, or body weight exercises. If you're new to strength training but are motivated to begin a program, try one of the many fitness applications that are available for download. For $.99, with a great app, you can turn your smartphone into a personal trainer.

Targeted Tips for Strength-Training Success

- If your attire for your big event reveals your arms, add 10 minutes per day of push-ups, tricep dips, and lateral raises to your regular strength-training workout. Do three sets of 15 to 20 repetitions per day.

- If you'll be showcasing your legs in shorts or a short dress, consider running the stairs or the stadium steps at the local high school. Stop and do a set of 15 calf raises at the bottom and top of each set.

- If you'll be wearing a swimsuit and want to tone your stomach and build shapely shoulders to balance out your physique, consider paddle boarding, kayaking, or tennis.

Remember, exercise is going to be a key factor in the results of your supercharged reset. Plan your days out in advance, put your workout on your calendar, and stick to the plan. We promise that the results will be worth it! Like the saying goes, no one has ever regretted that workout they just finished.

SUPERCHARGED RESET #1:
RESET YOUR WEIGHT IN 21 DAYS

If you're looking to lose a full clothing size or more, begin your supercharged reset three weeks out. A serious commitment to a twenty-one day program will help you reach your goal. This plan takes total dedication for total transformation. You can do it. Keep your eye on the prize. Mark your event date on your calendar and count down as the days go by.

First Ten Days:

- Two days of prep
- Three days of liquid cleansing
- Two days of postcleanse meals
- One more all-liquid day
- Two more days of whole-foods reset meals

Next Eleven Days:

- Six days of liquid meals combined with one whole-food meal
- Three days of liquid cleansing
- Two postcleanse days of juices, smoothies, salads, and light snacks

Let's get to it!

Days 1 and 2

These are your precleanse days to get ready for the upcoming all liquid days.

Reset Your Attitude and Your Mindset If you have not already done so, now is the time to pick your goal and visualize it with laser-sharp focus. Whether it's fitting into a piece of clothing or feeling like a million bucks when you see that old friend, identify your focus and reflect on this goal often.

Reset Your Energy Aim to cut out caffeine. However, if you aren't willing to let go of your caffeine addiction during the reset, switch to green tea or a low-acid, organic coffee variety. A few days into the program, you may find that your energy is so high that you don't need that added morning boost. Get ready to transform in the next twenty-one days.

Reset Your Metabolism You're eliminating processed foods and consuming more frequent meals to get your metabolism back on track.

Reset Your Taste Buds Begin each morning by drinking 1 cup of warm water with a big squeeze of fresh lemon. This morning ritual stimulates digestion and promotes alkalinity while bringing your taste buds back into balance to reduce cravings.

Reset Your Digestive System During these precleanse days, you're feeding your body plentiful amounts of fiber and chlorophyll-rich greens to get your digestive system moving things through and out more efficiently.

Reset Your Weight

> Day 1: Turn to page 66 and follow the meal plan for Two Days Before the Juice Cleanse.
>
> Day 2: Turn to page 67 and follow the meal plan for One Day Before the Juice Cleanse. You're only three weeks away from a slimmer, leaner you.

Reset Your Beauty Skin brushing, sauna sessions, or detox baths are all great ways to assist your body to begin cleaning impurities out of your system in order to maximize your benefits from this super-charged reset.

Reset Your Exercise Before eating anything, upon rising, do forty-five minutes of cardio at your moderate fat-burning pace (zone 2 or 60 to 70 percent of your max heart rate). You can go on a walk or use a piece of gym equipment leisurely to accomplish this.

Days 3, 4, and 5

These are juicing or smoothie days. Get ready for serious liquid nutrition.

Reset Your Attitude and Your Mindset At the end of each day or first thing in the morning before getting out of bed, celebrate your accomplishment of feeding your body great liquid nutrition while giving your digestive system a much-needed break. Acknowledge the strength of your willpower to resist the primal desire to chew.

Reset Your Energy The liquid portion of your supercharged reset may leave you sleeping better than ever before. Without the constant burden of breaking down food, you'll experience restful and restorative sleep.

Reset Your Metabolism Drink a juice or smoothie every few hours throughout the day to keep your metabolism going. Stay on top of drinking your juices/smoothies, even if you're not feeling hungry. If you skip a juice and end up starving, it becomes a challenge to return to a place of balance.

Reset Your Taste Buds These three days are like an intensive taste-bud boot camp that will kick your cravings to the curb. You're fueling your cells with enzymes and nutrients while flushing out any residual processed foods and chemicals. Upon completing the liquid phase of your supercharged reset, cravings will be a thing of the past.

Reset Your Digestive System Continue your morning ritual of warm water and lemon. During these three days, you're flooding your body with a bounty of fruits and vegetables in readily available liquid form, allowing your digestive system a much-enjoyed break and the opportunity to heal from past damage.

Reset Your Weight Turn to page 85 and follow the meal plans for the three-day juice cleanse. You should be able to ease into these liquid days with little problem after following two days of the precleanse. After three days of liquid nutrition, you'll eliminate excess water weight, drop a few pounds, and feel motivated to achieve your goal.

Reset Your Beauty Do a dry skin brush daily plus two sauna sessions or detox baths during these three days. Indulge yourself with one of the natural facials that best fit your needs (see pages 133–136). Get to bed early and take naps whenever possible during your liquid days. Sleep offers your body the best opportunity to repair cells and recuperate from life's daily demands.

Reset Your Exercise

Day 3: Before your first juice or smoothie, do forty minutes of cardio at your moderate fat-burning pace (50 to 60 percent of your max heart rate).

Day 4: Do Pilates or yoga for at least forty-five minutes.

Day 5: Before your first juice or smoothie, do forty minutes of cardio at your moderate fat-burning pace (50 to 60 percent of your max heart rate).

Days 6 and 7

Time to add back in solid foods after three fabulous days of all liquid.

Reset Your Attitude and Your Mindset Throw away all negative thoughts. You are doing amazingly well. After these days of plant-based, organic foods, you should experience clarity and energy. Choose to release negative emotions. You can treat this as a mental exercise, or you can write down any negative thoughts that still weigh you down and then shred, burn, or stomp on the paper. Try this for a sense of immediate gratification.

Reset Your Energy By now, you should be experiencing the vitality-giving benefits of eating high-quality, pure, organic foods. Take note of how your energy has improved from the time you started this reset until today.

Reset Your Metabolism Feeding your body real food that it understands how to process will keep your metabolism running as it should.

Reset Your Taste Buds Continue your morning lemon water ritual. You have probably noticed by now that beginning your day with warm water and lemon makes it easier to make healthy choices all day.

Reset Your Digestive System On these solid food days, post-juicing and smoothie days, you should feel relief from any digestion issues or bloating you had pre-reset. If you still have symptoms, consider the herbal teas we discussed on page 75.

Reset Your Weight Turn to page 98 and follow the meal plans for the first two postcleanse days in chapter 5. This will extend the benefits of your liquid cleanse days and continue to flush toxins.

Reset Your Beauty Continue dry brushing. If at all possible, enjoy a sauna session or detox bath to keep your pores open and clear.

Reset Your Exercise

Day 6: Before your first meal, do forty minutes of cardio at moderate fat-burning pace.

Day 7: Rest day or outside activity with a friend. Go on a walk or a moderate hike or bike ride. Golf or play tennis or beach volleyball.

Day 8

Today you jump right back into a one-day, all-liquid fast. It should be easy now that your system is clean and your cravings are gone. Get ready to glow.

Reset Your Attitude and Your Mindset Yesterday you eliminated your negative thoughts. Now it's time to deepen your connection to what you wish to bring into your life in order to fill the space you freed.

If you released negative self-talk, replace it with affirmations. If you released attachment to how others judge you, replace it with dedication to treating yourself with kindness. Whatever it was that you let go of, now is the time to invite and welcome in its better counterpart.

Reset Your Energy Today is an energy-boosting day. This one-day fast comes at the perfect time to recharge. Because you have been eating clean food and your diet has been free from foods that would typically bog down your energy and make transitioning to liquid a challenge, today you'll notice that you have more energy than your first all-liquid day last week.

Reset Your Metabolism After juice and smoothies only today, your metabolism will be ready to burn through tomorrow's meals quickly.

Reset Your Taste Buds All-liquid days flood your body with nutrients and enzymes that will leave you craving pure and fresh foods on the days that follow.

Reset Your Digestive System Today is a great example of how embarking upon a single day of abstaining from food can be just the break your digestive system needs to heal and reboot.

Reset Your Weight Select from any of the juice or smoothie recipes in this book. Aim for six juices per day or four smoothies. If you're combining both juice and smoothies, we suggest two smoothies and three juices.

Reset Your Beauty Continue dry brushing today. This evening enjoy a detox bath or sauna session. Because it's a fasting day, try to get to bed as early as possible or to sneak in a nap. Getting adequate sleep is essential on fasting days in order for your body to reap maximum benefits.

Reset Your Exercise It's time to increase your fat-burning cardio (50 to 60 percent of your max heart rate) to fifty minutes per session this week. Remember, we suggest you do this cardio first thing in the morning. If that is not possible for you, make sure you get this session on your calendar for another time during the day.

Days 9 and 10

These are two days of meals before you transition into smoothies and juices and one meal per day. If possible, prepare these meals in advance.

Reset Your Attitude and Your Mindset Revisit the reset your attitude and your mindset practice from day 8. Stay committed to the same practice for days 9 and 10. Repeating your goals over and over brings them closer to reality. If you have ever considered creating a vision board, now is the time to get that started. Think big and begin turning your vision into your reality.

Reset Your Energy Pay attention to how you feel after meals. Take note of any surges or slumps in your energy and adjust your future meals accordingly. This is your reset! If there are certain meals that do not make you feel your best, feel free to change them out with another option from the recipes in this book.

Reset Your Metabolism Remember to continue drinking at least 64 ounces per day of good-quality water to keep your metabolism and systems of elimination working at their peak.

Reset Your Taste Buds Continue your warm water and lemon ritual. Remember, this morning ritual stimulates digestion and promotes alkalinity while enhancing elimination and decreasing cravings.

Reset Your Digestive System If you used herbal teas yesterday, hopefully you feel the benefits today. Continue to drink lots of water between your juices in order to keep your cells hydrated and electrolytes balanced.

Reset Your Weight Enjoy a smoothie or juice for breakfast and choose any of the meals and snacks found in this book for lunch, snack, and dinner.

Reset Your Beauty Do skin brushing and a natural exfoliating treatment. For extra silky skin, slather coconut oil on your skin for a natural and chemical-free moisturizer.

Reset Your Exercise Continue with daily fifty-minute-long fat-burning sessions.

Days 11, 12, 13, 14, 15, and 16

During these days, you'll consume all liquids until dinner. Juicing until dinner allows your body to continue with the removal of toxins and flushing of excess weight, while you still enjoy an evening meal. If you have a work meeting or lunch with a friend, you may switch to having your one meal of the day be lunch instead of dinner. If you do so, replace dinner with a smoothie or juice.

Reset Your Attitude and Your Mindset Challenge yourself to cleanse yourself of excess technology for these four days. Instead of jumping on your phone to check email or status updates while waiting in line at the grocery store, practice being still and mindful of all that is happening around you. This simple modification to your day can increase your energy and sense of well-being. Try it!

Reset Your Energy Your energy will soar during these days. You'll notice that you can feel completely satisfied from liquids alone.

Reset Your Metabolism Each day, you're essentially embarking upon a fifteen-hour or longer fast. Your fasting hours will be fueled by nature's best offerings, and your body will take on the task of breaking down your evening meal with ease.

Reset Your Taste Buds You'll find that after feeding your body delicious smoothies and juices all day, you'll crave the healthiest of foods for your dinner.

Reset Your Digestive System Your digestive system will be operating at its optimal level. The combination of chlorophyll-rich smoothies and juices and a fiber-rich final meal are the ideal recipe for awesome digestive health.

Reset Your Weight

Breakfast: Juice or smoothie

Snack: Juice or smoothie

Lunch: Juice or smoothie

Dinner: Choose any meal from this book

Reset Your Beauty Continue dry brushing. During these days, use the extra time you freed up by cutting out unneeded technology to enjoy two detox baths or sauna sessions and at least one facial and two body scrubs.

Reset Your Exercise Time to increase your fat-burning cardio to sixty minutes per day. Remember to listen to your body and to pace yourself accordingly.

Days 17, 18, and 19

You're five days away from completing this supercharged reset! You have already come so far and your big day is right around the corner. These next three days are your final all-liquid days. By now, you know which your favorite juices and smoothies are. Stick to those for these three days, but make sure you're getting plenty of greens. You're also welcome to add a plant-based protein powder (page 108) to your smoothies if it feels right for you.

Reset Your Attitude and Your Mindset Accept all parts of yourself and your life. If you have beat yourself up for as long as you can remember about your thighs touching or your stomach not being as flat as you would hope, forgive those parts today. Accept and embrace how beautiful, vibrant, and healthy you are.

Reset Your Energy By now, you probably feel better than ever. At this point of the program, many people begin to feel like they can live on much less sleep. Enjoy your newfound energy, but continue to aim for seven to eight hours of sleep each night.

Reset Your Metabolism Your body is now completely clear of processed foods, additives, and chemicals that may have previously interfered with your digestion.

Reset Your Taste Buds Relish in how wonderfully sweet the season's best fruits and vegetables taste to you at this point. If post-reset, you lose this sense of satisfaction from fruits and vegetables, take that as your signal that it's time to get back to a mini reset.

Reset Your Digestive System Your morning lemon water continues to be an important part of your daily ritual for digestive health.

Reset Your Weight Do the three-day juice cleanse from chapter 4.

Reset Your Beauty Continue with skin brushing. Moisturize with organic coconut oil. Drink lots of water.

Reset Your Exercise Do forty-five to sixty minutes of fat-burning cardio. Listen to your body to determine length.

Drink Water!

Avoid the mistake of decreasing your water consumption before an event. It's well documented that your metabolism slows down when calorie consumption decreases too drastically, and, as a result, your body stores fat in case it needs it later. This same pattern applies to water. If your body is deprived of water, it'll hold on to the water it has in case it needs to survive a long period without water. This leads to water retention, stagnant energy, and toxins being stored. On the other hand, the more you flood your body with high-quality, filtered water, the more easily your body releases excess water and eliminates toxins in doing so. Drinking loads of water before a big event helps your skin glow and helps eliminate bloat.

Days 20 and 21

Two days to go!! You'll ease back into solid foods by integrating salads and light snacks. Approach your big event looking and feeling your best!

Reset Your Attitude and Your Mindset Affirm yourself and tell everyone who will listen how great you feel and what you have accomplished. Aim to surround yourself with people who support and love your best self. No one has the power to bring you down, but it's much easier to live your best and healthiest life when the people around you support your awesomeness.

Reset Your Energy Sugar-, carb-, and caffeine-induced peaks and valleys of your energy should be a distant memory by now.

Reset Your Metabolism Know that you're able to listen to your body and judge when you're truly hungry and when you're thinking of food out of boredom or to fill an emotional need. Your metabolism is back in working order now that you're free from hormone-filled foods and other chemically manipulated foods that interfere with your body's signals.

Reset Your Taste Buds On these final days of your supercharged reset, pay attention to how delicious real food tastes. Make a conscious decision to stick with eating real food only. This alone will greatly improve your health.

Reset Your Digestive System Now that your system is working efficiently, you can easily tell how various foods influence your digestion. Vow not to ignore the many messages your body sends.

Reset Your Weight

> Breakfast: Green juice or green smoothie
>
> Lunch: Any green salad from this book
>
> Snack: Any snack from this book
>
> Dinner: Juice or smoothie of choice

Reset Your Beauty Enjoy your facial on day 20. On day 21, indulge in a great body scrub, followed by coconut oil moisturizer. Optional sauna session.

Reset Your Exercise Do sixty minutes of fat-burning cardio. You have come this far. Make sure you fit in these last two sweaty sessions.

Bravo!!! You completed your twenty-one day supercharged reset and will present your best self at your big event.

SUPERCHARGED RESET #2:
RESET YOUR HEALTH IN 10 DAYS

You're about to embark upon ten days to change. Dedicate yourself to this plan for ten days and you'll feel and look your absolute best in time for your big day.

The Supercharged Reset Plan:

- Two days of accelerated preparation
- Six days of juices or smoothies
- Two days of liquid meals for breakfast, meal of your choice for lunch, and a liquid dinner

Let's do it!

Days 1 and 2

These two days are about getting you ready for your upcoming six-day juice and smoothie cleanse. Following these two prep days will help you transition into the all-liquid days with ease.

Reset Your Attitude and Your Mindset When you choose to make yourself a priority, there are no limits to what you can accomplish! What can you eliminate from your life to create more time for yourself each day? Can you to take a hiatus from social media, give up a TV program, wake up an hour earlier each day, or give up a social engagement?

Reset Your Energy You may experience a dip in your energy these first few days as you wean off of sugars, caffeine, and food additives. Know that it's temporary and will pass.

Reset Your Metabolism By eliminating processed foods from your diet, your metabolism recalibrates to its optimal level.

Reset Your Taste Buds Begin each morning by drinking 1 cup of warm water with a big squeeze of fresh lemon. This morning ritual stimulates digestion and promotes alkalinity while enhancing elimination and decreasing cravings.

Reset Your Digestive System Sip on herbal detox teas throughout the day (page 75) to begin waking up your cleansing organs.

Reset Your Weight

Day 1: Turn to page 66 and follow the meal plan for Two Days Before the Juice Cleanse.

Day 2: Turn to page 67 and follow the meal plan for One Day Before the Juice Cleanse.

Reset Your Beauty Skin brush daily and do a body scrub on day 2. After showering or bathing, moisturize with coconut oil.

Reset Your Exercise Do forty-five minutes of fat-burning cardio upon rising, on an empty stomach. If you feel up to it, you may opt to add a second forty-five-minute cardio session on day 2.

Need a Pick-Me-Up?

If your energy lags and you need an extra boost to help you power through your cardio sessions, feel free to incorporate antioxidant-rich green tea for instant energy.

Days 3, 4, 5, 6, 7, and 8

You're about to embark upon six spectacular days of juices and smoothies. Make sure that you have all of your ingredients and get ready to feel fantastic!

Reset Your Attitude and Your Mindset Six days of juicing is a big endeavor. Stay focused on your goal and visualize how great you'll feel upon completing this reset. You can do this!

Reset Your Energy If you experience fatigue or any other "healing crisis," visit page 73 for tips to help you to get through the symptoms quickly. Once you do, your energy levels will soar.

Reset Your Metabolism You're resetting your metabolism by consuming a juice or smoothie every few hours throughout the day. Do not skip juices.

Reset Your Taste Buds The juices and smoothies that you're enjoying are designed to feed your cells the nutrients and enzymes they most need. Upon completing the cleanse, you'll crave nature's purest and most nutrient-dense foods.

Reset Your Digestive System These six days provide your digestive system a well-deserved rest, which allows your system to eliminate stored-up toxins and repair past damage.

Reset Your Weight Follow the juice cleanse from chapter 4 for six days.

Reset Your Beauty Skin brush daily. Moisturize with coconut oil after showering or bathing. Aim to take three detox baths or sauna sessions over these six days and to enjoy two or three body treatments or facials.

Reset Your Exercise Do forty-five minutes of fat-burning exercise, preferably upon rising. Aim to add an extra session of cardio on two of these six days.

Strength Training

Continue your normal strength-training program, if you have one. If you don't have one, we advise not starting one at this time for two reasons: (1) you'll be hungrier, and (2) your muscles may retain extra water when you first start a strength regimen.

You'll get the most immediate visible results from your cardio. For this reason, we suggest that you focus on this if you don't have an existing strength-training program or if you do not have enough time for both a cardio and a strength routine.

Days 9 and 10

These two postcleanse days combine juices or smoothies with whole food meals in order to ease you back into eating solid foods while sustaining the benefits you have achieved.

Reset Your Attitude and Your Mindset You have proven to yourself that you have stellar willpower. Keep this confidence with you and tap into it whenever temptation is in your path.

Reset Your Energy Your energy levels should be steady now that you have eliminated energy-zapping processed foods, sugars, and additives.

Reset Your Metabolism Your metabolism is reset to want food throughout the day. Even if you're not feeling too hungry, avoid skipping meals or juices. You can opt for smaller portions, but continue to feed your body every few hours in order to keep your metabolism high.

Reset Your Taste Buds You have eliminated cravings for high-fat and sugar-laden foods.

Reset Your Digestive System If you have any bloating or discomfort as you add food back in, try an herbal tea. For some options, visit page 75.

Reset Your Weight For breakfast, make any smoothie or juice recipe from this book that contains greens. Choose any lunch and snack recipe from chapter 8, and for dinner, choose any smoothie or juice recipe.

Reset Your Beauty On day 9, enjoy your favorite facial and body scrub (see page 133).

Reset Your Exercise On these last two days, do forty-five to sixty minutes of fat-burning, sweat-inducing, toxin-flushing cardio upon rising. Remember, your first workout is in the morning, upon rising, on an empty stomach. If you feel up to the challenge, add a second forty-five-minute session on day 10.

Bravo!!! You have completed your ten-day supercharged reset.

SUPERCHARGED RESET #3:
RESET AND REFRESH IN 3 DAYS

If you follow a healthy, clean eating plan and are pretty happy with your weight, but still have the desire for a mini reset in order to be at your absolute best for a special occasion, the three-day supercharged reset is the plan for you.

The Supercharged Reset Plan:

- One prep day of two liquid meals, one snack, and one solid meal
- Two days of juices and smoothies

Here we go!

Days 1–3

These three days are about quick transformation. Your energy will be boosted, your eyes will be brighter, and your pants will be a wee bit looser—all in just three days.

Reset Your Attitude and Your Mindset

The quickest way to give yourself a mental makeover that is guaranteed to improve your mindset is to practice gratitude. There are two parts to your three-day gratitude practice:

1. Take out a piece of paper and list everything you can think of that you're grateful for. Include big things like your family and your health, and little things like finding a good parking spot at the store today or finding that thing that has been missing forever. Make a special point to include the unique things that bring you unexpected joy like your favorite song, the amusing billboard you passed by today, or the way your most comfy lounge pants feel when you put them on after a long day. Read this list each morning and evening and add to it. The more time you spend with your list, the more it grows as you find more and more reasons to be grateful!

2. Sometimes people complain simply for the sake of complaining. It's a way to fill in gaps of silence. Now that you have written your gratitude list and realize that there is so much for you to be grateful for, commit to focus on the positive and indulge yourself in three days of NO negativity. For these three days, vow to abstain from complaining. You may not be aware of how many negative things leave your mouth each day until you make a conscious decision to avoid saying anything negative. When you eliminate negative chatter, miracles can happen—somehow the negative things that you didn't complain about go away on their own.

Reset Your Energy In three days, you'll have more energy and will wake up on the morning of your event feeling refreshed.

Reset Your Metabolism These three days will kick your metabolism back up to high gear, leaving you burning calories efficiently.

Reset Your Taste Buds You'll be amazed at how, in three short days, you can greatly diminish cravings for salty and sugary foods by feeding your body the nutrients that it really needs for vibrant health.

Reset Your Digestive System Because this is a short reset, you want to be sure to get things moving right away. If necessary, you may consider an herbal tea (see page 75) to support your detox.

Reset Your Weight

Day 1: This is an accelerated prep day for your two-day juice cleanse. Have a juice or smoothie for breakfast, a meal of your choice for lunch, a snack each day, and a juice or smoothie for dinner.

Days 2 and 3: Turn to page 85 and follow the meal plan for the first two days of the juice cleanse from chapter 4.

Reset Your Beauty Skin brush daily and apply coconut oil moisturizer after showering or bathing.

Days 1 and 3: Natural body scrub—we suggest the coffee ground scrub on page 137 to increase circulation and decrease cellulite. Try to do at least one detox bath or sauna session and one facial treatment.

Reset Your Exercise One hour of sweat-inducing yet low-intensity cardio upon rising. If dropping a few pounds is part of your three-day goal, add an extra forty-minute fat-burning session at another time during the day. Do not try to go a straight hour and forty minutes. It's important to split these cardio sessions for best results and so that the sessions don't zap your energy.

Bravo!!! You completed your three-day supercharged reset!

Whether you embark on the twenty-one-day, ten-day, or three-day reset, fully commit to following the plan! Remember to do your grocery shopping in advance and to clear your kitchen of any foods that could derail your success. If you should fall off the wagon, promise yourself you'll jump right back on. In addition to the aesthetic changes you'll see, you'll feel better and will have more energy. Walk into your big event with the confidence that you look as good on the outside as you feel on the inside. Enjoy yourself!

eight

THE
RECIPES

"The doctor of the future will no longer treat the human frame with drugs, but rather will cure and prevent disease with nutrition."

—Thomas Edison

All of the recipes mentioned earlier in this book are contained here. We've organized them into categories, beginning with juices and smoothies. The meals are organized into breakfast, lunch, dinner, and snack, and we also have some soup and homemade vinaigrette recipes for you. Each recipe is simple to prepare and uses easily obtained ingredients. Most can be made ahead and then eaten cold or reheated.

GREEN JUICES

The juices will be made in a juicer, *not* a blender. If you don't have a juicer, but do have a Vitamix or a blender, skip to the green smoothie section (page 172). If you have a juicer, please use that for the juice-cleanse portion of the Juice Cleanse Reset Diet, as you'll have faster results while juicing. The fiber is removed from the fruit and vegetables in the juicing process, while in the Vitamix or blender, it's left in the finished product, making a smoothie rather than a juice. These juice recipes won't taste the same or have the correct consistency if you try to make them in your blender.

These green juices have a combination of vegetables and fruit for maximum nutrition. They're the building blocks of your cleanse and a great addition to your diet every day. The leafy green veggies give these juices color, minerals, and vitamins, and the fruit adds natural sweetness to keep them tasty. Once you are accustomed to the basic flavors of these juices and smoothies, experiment with adding more greens and less fruit. Preparing juices and smoothies is not an exact science. Variables such as the type of juicer or blender and the ripeness of the produce will yield varying textures and quantities of juice. Feel free to adjust the recipes as desired. Minor tweaks will not impact your results.

Lemon Green Juice

This juice is great first thing in the morning, as the lemon gets your metabolism started and the leafy greens provide essential vitamins and minerals to energize you for the day. MAKES 16 OUNCES

$\frac{1}{2}$ lemon
1 cup spinach
$\frac{1}{2}$ head romaine lettuce
1 cup chopped cucumber
1 large Granny Smith apple, sliced

Juice the lemon using a manual citrus juicer. Juice the remaining ingredients in a juicer, and then combine with the lemon juice. Store in an airtight glass container in the refrigerator for up to 24 hours.

Mango-Kale Juice

This is a green juice that doesn't taste green. The mango adds antioxidants and sweet flavor, while the nutrients in the kale and apples help detoxify the liver and fight free radicals. MAKES 16 OUNCES

2 bunches kale
2 mangoes, pitted
1 large Granny Smith apple, sliced

Juice all of the ingredients in a juicer. Store in an airtight glass container in the refrigerator for up to 24 hours.

Green Ginger Juice

The addition of ginger to this green concoction boosts immunity and aids in digestion, while adding a zing of flavor. MAKES 16 OUNCES

1 bunch kale
4 stalks celery
1 cup spinach
1 cucumber, chopped
2 Granny Smith apples, sliced
1 ($^1/_2$-inch) piece ginger root

Juice all of the ingredients in a juicer. Store in an airtight glass container in the refrigerator for up to 24 hours.

Green Carrot Juice

A sweet concoction that boosts your immune system, helps reduce inflammation, and flushes excess water from your system while loading you up with antioxidants. MAKES 16 OUNCES

$^1/_2$ lemon
3 carrots
1 cucumber, chopped
2 handfuls dandelion greens
$^1/_2$ cup cubed pineapple

Juice the lemon using a manual citrus juicer. Juice the remaining ingredients in a juicer, and then combine with the lemon juice. Store in an airtight glass container in the refrigerator for up to 24 hours.

Red Ginger Juice

This juice is a real energy boost, and it's great when you need a pick-me-up or when you need to fuel a workout. The fruit provides energy, while the beet increases endurance, and the celery and fennel push out toxins. MAKES 16 OUNCES

1 lime
1 beet
1 Granny Smith apple, sliced
1 pear, sliced
4 stalks celery
1 fennel bulb, chopped
1 ($1/4$-inch) piece ginger root
1 ($1/4$-inch) piece turmeric root

Juice the lime using a manual citrus juicer. Juice the remaining ingredients in a juicer, and then combine with the lime juice. Store in an airtight glass container in the refrigerator for up to 24 hours.

Green Pineapple Juice

A great way to get your kids to drink their greens. The pineapple helps with digestion and reduces inflammation, while the greens add vitamins and nutrients. MAKES 16 OUNCES

1 bunch kale
1 bunch spinach, or 2 cups loose baby spinach
1 bunch romaine
$1/2$ pineapple, cubed

Juice all of the ingredients in a juicer. Store in an airtight glass container in the refrigerator for up to 24 hours.

Wild Green Juice

This is a lighter version of Green Pineapple Juice (page 168). The cucumber, celery, and dandelion act to hydrate while flushing out toxins.

MAKES 16 OUNCES

> $^1/_2$ pineapple, cubed
> 4 stalks celery
> 1 cucumber, chopped
> 4 leaves kale
> Handful of wild greens (such as dandelion)
> 1 ($^1/_2$-inch) piece ginger root

Juice all of the ingredients in a juicer. Store in an airtight glass container in the refrigerator for up to 24 hours.

Spinach-Pineapple-Mint Juice

The mint in this juice ties together the sweet pineapple and tart green apple so well that you won't even notice the spinach. **MAKES 16 OUNCES**

> $^1/_2$ lemon
> 3 cups spinach
> 2 Granny Smith apples, sliced
> 2 cups cubed pineapple
> 8 mint leaves

Juice the lemon using a manual citrus juicer. Juice the remaining ingredients in a juicer, and then combine with the lemon juice. Store in an airtight glass container in the refrigerator for up to 24 hours.

Kale-Basil Juice

A savory blend that will have you dreaming of Rome. Kale, basil, apples, celery, and fennel combine with coconut water and spices to detoxify and repair skin cells. **MAKES 16 OUNCES**

1 cup kale
1 cup basil
2 Granny Smith apples, sliced
3 stalks celery
1 fennel bulb, chopped
1 (¼-inch) piece ginger root
1 (¼-inch) piece turmeric root
1 cup coconut water

Juice all of the ingredients except the coconut water in a juicer. Combine with the coconut water. Store in an airtight glass container in the refrigerator for up to 24 hours.

Carrot-Beet Juice

This juice is surprisingly sweet and refreshing for a vegetable blend. It's supercleansing and chock-full of beta-carotene. **MAKES 16 OUNCES**

1 large carrot
1 large red beet, chopped
1 red apple, sliced
1 stalk celery
1 (½-inch) piece ginger root

Juice all of the ingredients in a juicer. Store in an airtight glass container in the refrigerator for up to 24 hours.

FRUIT JUICES

These juices contain mainly fruit and are a bit sweeter than the green juices. They have a higher sugar content than the green juices and should be limited to one or two juices per day on the cleanse. Drinking one when you have an energy slump or before a workout can be especially helpful.

Apple-Ginger Juice

A zesty update to apple juice. A sweet source of immunity-boosting vitamins and minerals. **MAKES 16 OUNCES**

> 1 lemon
> 3 apples, sliced
> 1 (¹/₂-inch) piece ginger root

Juice the lemon using a manual citrus juicer. Juice the remaining ingredients in a juicer, and then combine with the lemon juice. Store in an airtight glass container in the refrigerator for up to 24 hours.

Apple-Berry Juice

A blend of berry flavors sweetens any palate. The antioxidants in the berries will help fight free radicals and rejuvenate your beauty in no time. **MAKES 16 OUNCES**

> 2 apples, sliced
> 1 cup strawberries, hulled
> 1 cup blueberries

Juice all of the ingredients in a juicer. Store in an airtight glass container in the refrigerator for up to 24 hours.

Ginger-Pear Juice

Pear, citrus, and ginger combine to create a powerful immunity-boosting juice, full of vitamin C. **MAKES 16 OUNCES**

> 1 tangerine
> 1 lemon
> 1 large pear, sliced
> 1 ($\frac{1}{2}$-inch) piece ginger root
> Pinch of cayenne (optional)

Juice the tangerine and lemon using a manual citrus juicer. Juice the pear and ginger in a juicer, and then combine with the citrus juices. Mix in the cayenne if you want an extra kick. Store in an airtight glass container in the refrigerator for up to 24 hours.

GREEN SMOOTHIES

Time to break out the blender and whip up some smoothies. Although the bits of fiber in the drinks will make them thicker, they'll also keep you full longer. For smoothies, you can use banana or avocado to add creaminess and flavor. Please note that the strength and capability of your blender will affect the consistency of your smoothie. If it seems too thick, you can add water, coconut water, or even some of your homemade almond or hemp milk. If you use all fresh ingredients (no frozen fruit), add ½ cup of ice, if the recipe doesn't already include it, to make your smoothie cold.

When you're on the juice-cleanse portion of the reset diet, it's best to use a juicer, if you have one, and follow the juice recipes. If you don't have a juicer, use the smoothie recipes that follow in your Vitamix or blender.

Green Banana Smoothie

This creamy blend of banana, spinach, and kale is combined with apple to deliver an energizing, nutrient-dense, fiber-rich, and satisfying smoothie. **MAKES 16 OUNCES**

1 large handful spinach (about 1 cup)
1 large handful kale (about 1 cup)
1 banana, peeled
1 red apple, cored and sliced
$^1/_2$ cup water
$^1/_2$ cup ice

Combine all of the ingredients in a high-speed blender and blend until smooth. Store in an airtight glass container in the refrigerator for up to 24 hours.

Green Almond Smoothie

This protein-rich green smoothie will satisfy your sweet tooth while sustaining your energy for hours. **MAKES 16 OUNCES**

1 large handful spinach (about 1 cup)
1 cup Almond Milk (page 181)
2 pears, cored and sliced
1 frozen banana, peeled

Combine all of the ingredients in a high-speed blender and blend until smooth. Store in an airtight glass container in the refrigerator for up to 24 hours.

Black and Green Smoothie

This speckled combination of pineapple, blackberry, and spinach boosts your immune system while delivering a healthy dose of iron, protein, and antioxidants. **MAKES 16 OUNCES**

> 2 handfuls spinach (about 2 cups)
> $1/2$ pineapple, cubed
> $3/4$ cup blackberries

Combine all of the ingredients in a high-speed blender and blend until smooth. Store in an airtight glass container in the refrigerator for up to 24 hours.

Green Berry Smoothie

You won't even notice the taste of kale in this berry, apple, and carrot blend. From increasing energy to detoxifying the liver and fighting free radicals, this smoothie does it all. **MAKES 16 OUNCES**

> $1/2$ bunch kale, chopped (about 1 cup)
> 1 handful mixed baby greens (about 1 cup)
> 1 carrot, chopped
> 1 green apple, cored and sliced
> 1 cup raspberries
> $1/2$ cup water
> $1/2$ cup ice

Combine all of the ingredients in a high-speed blender and blend until smooth. Store in an airtight glass container in the refrigerator for up to 24 hours.

Green Energy Smoothie

Antioxidant-rich green tea delivers an energy boost in this refreshing blend of melon, spinach, and cucumber. This will also help you shed excess water and rid your body of toxins. **MAKES 16 OUNCES**

$1/2$ lemon
1 cup spinach
$1/2$ cucumber, seeded and peeled
1 cup honeydew melon, cubed
1 cup organic green tea

Juice the lemon using a manual citrus juicer. Add the lemon juice and the remaining ingredients to a high-speed blender and blend until smooth. Store in an airtight glass container in the refrigerator for up to 24 hours.

FRUIT SMOOTHIES

These smoothies are composed mostly of fruit. Although fruit made into a smoothie contains fiber and therefore slows your body's sugar absorption, you should still limit these smoothies to one or two per day while on the juice-cleanse portion of the reset diet. Midmorning, midafternoon, or preworkout are the best times to have a fruit smoothie.

Banana-Berry Smoothie

Banana serves as a creamy complement to berries. It boosts the absorption of antioxidants and phytonutrients and helps your skin stay soft and supple. **MAKES 16 OUNCES**

continued >

Banana-Berry Smoothie, continued

> 1 large orange
> $^1/_4$ cup blueberries
> $^1/_2$ cup raspberries
> 1 kiwi, peeled
> 1 frozen banana, peeled
> $^1/_2$ cup ice

Juice the orange using a manual citrus juicer. Add the juice and the remaining ingredients to a high-speed blender and blend until smooth. Store in an airtight glass container in the refrigerator for up to 24 hours.

Strawberry-Banana Smoothie

High in vitamin C and potassium, this delicious blend of strawberries and banana will make you think you're having dessert while you're boosting your immune system. MAKES 16 OUNCES

> 2 cups strawberries, hulled
> 1 frozen banana, peeled
> 1 cup ice

Combine all of the ingredients in a high-speed blender and blend until smooth. Store in an airtight glass container in the refrigerator for up to 24 hours.

Honeydew-Orange Smoothie

This smoothie has an abundance of summer fruit and melon to aid in cell regeneration, rid the body of toxins, and reduce inflammation. MAKES 16 OUNCES

> 1 orange
> 1 cup cubed honeydew melon

$^1/_2$ peach, peeled and pitted
$^1/_2$ cup cubed pineapple
1 cup ice

Juice the orange using a manual citrus juicer. Add the juice and the remaining ingredients to a high-speed blender and blend until smooth. Store in an airtight glass container in the refrigerator for up to 24 hours.

Kiwi-Berry Smoothie

Kiwi, blueberry, and banana combine to boost your beauty quotient. With phytonutrients and antioxidants, your skin will glow and be refreshed. MAKES 16 OUNCES

3 kiwis, peeled
2 cups blueberries
1 green apple, cored and sliced
$^1/_2$ cup ice

Combine all the ingredients in a high-speed blender and blend until smooth. Store in an airtight glass container in the refrigerator for up to 24 hours.

Greensicle Smoothie

Remember eating Creamsicles when you were a kid? The combination of creamy vanilla ice cream and orange Popsicle was so tasty and satisfying. This grown-up version is made with almond milk, oranges, and kale—a healthy version of that childhood treat in a glass.
MAKES 16 OUNCES

1 orange
1 cup chopped kale
$^1/_2$ cup Almond Milk (page 181)
1 cup ice cubes

continued >

Greensicle Smoothie, continued

Juice the orange using a manual citrus juicer. Add the juice and the remaining ingredients to a high-speed blender and blend until smooth. Store in an airtight glass container in the refrigerator for up to 24 hours.

Cherry-Berry Smoothie

The flavors of cherries and raspberries combine to boost metabolism, curb appetite, and fight free radicals. **MAKES 16 OUNCES**

> $^1/_2$ cup fresh cherries, pitted
> $^1/_2$ cucumber, peeled and seeded
> 1 apple, cored and sliced
> $^1/_2$ cup fresh or frozen raspberries
> $^1/_2$ cup ice

Combine all of the ingredients in a high-speed blender and blend until smooth. Store in an airtight glass container in the refrigerator for up to 24 hours.

Pineapple-Banana Smoothie

This tropical treat combines pineapple, banana, and coconut to give you a boost of potassium and bromelain, which increases skin hydration while reducing inflammation. **MAKES 16 OUNCES**

> 2 cups cubed pineapple
> $1^1/_2$ frozen bananas, peeled
> $^1/_2$ cup coconut water

Combine all of the ingredients in a high-speed blender and blend until smooth. Store in an airtight glass container in the refrigerator for up to 24 hours.

ALKALIZERS

Alkalizers will help you reach that slightly alkaline state we discussed in chapter 3. These juices are lighter than the others, slightly sweet, and super refreshing! These juices will store for a day or two longer than the juices and smoothies above.

Cucumber-Watermelon Juice

Nothing says summer more than watermelon. This alkalizing blend of cucumber, watermelon, and lime is cool and refreshing.

MAKES 16 OUNCES

$1/2$ lime
1 cucumber, peeled and seeded
2 cups cubed watermelon
$1/2$ cup ice cubes

Juice the lime using a manual citrus juicer. Juice the remaining ingredients in a juicer, and then combine with the lime juice. Alternately, add the lime juice and the remaining ingredients to a high-speed blender and blend until smooth. Store in an airtight glass container in the refrigerator for up to 36 hours.

Spicy Lemonade

This juice will boost your metabolism, help alkalize you, and curb your appetite. Lemonade with a kick! **MAKES 16 OUNCES**

1 lemon
12 ounces water
2 tablespoons raw agave
Cayenne pepper

continued >

Spicy Lemonade, continued

Juice the lemon using a manual citrus juicer. Combine the lemon juice, water, and agave, and then add cayenne pepper to taste. Store in an airtight glass container in the refrigerator for up to 36 hours.

Cucumber-Apple Juice

Cucumber, apple, and ginger give you a low-calorie, refreshing treat that will keep you craving more. The ginger adds an immunity-boosting zesty flavor. MAKES 16 OUNCES

    1 cucumber, chopped
    2 apples, sliced
    1 (½-inch) piece ginger root

Juice all of the ingredients in a juicer. Store in an airtight glass container in the refrigerator for up to 36 hours.

Coco Kale Juice

This refreshing blend of pears, coconut water, and kale will have you dreaming of the tropics while you increase your energy and detoxify your liver. MAKES 16 OUNCES

    1 lime
    1 handful kale
    1½ cups coconut water
    2 pears, sliced

Juice the lime using a manual citrus juicer. Juice the remaining ingredients in a juicer, and then combine with the lime juice. Store in an airtight glass container in the refrigerator for up to 36 hours.

MILKS

Although they are called *milks*, none of these juices contain any dairy. They are made from nuts or hemp seeds, and are high in protein and supersatisfying. While you're on the juice-cleanse portion of the reset diet, you'll drink a milk each night as your final meal. The combination of protein and healthy fats will help you sleep like a baby.

Almond Milk

This delicious nut milk will have you swearing off dairy forever. Full of protein, essential minerals, and healthy fats, this is the perfect protein shake. **MAKES 16 OUNCES**

> $^1/_2$ cup raw almonds, soaked in water for 6 to 8 hours, then drained
> $1^1/_2$ cups water
> 1 teaspoon vanilla extract
> $^1/_2$ teaspoon cinnamon
> 1 tablespoon raw agave, or 2 Medjool dates, pitted

Combine all of the ingredients in a high-speed blender and blend until smooth. Strain through a strainer or a chinois. Store in an airtight glass container in the refrigerator for up to 36 hours.

Cashew Milk

This is so tasty you'll think you're eating something bad for you rather than a great source of protein and potassium. **MAKES 16 OUNCES**

> $^2/_3$ cup raw cashew nuts, soaked in water for 4 hours, then drained
> 2 cups water
> 1 cup ice
> 1 Medjool date, pitted, or 1 teaspoon raw agave
> 2 frozen bananas, peeled

continued >

Cashew Milk, continued

> **2 tablespoons raw cacao powder (optional)**
> **1 teaspoon cinnamon**
> **A pinch of Celtic sea salt**

Combine all of the ingredients in a high-speed blender and blend until smooth. Store in an airtight glass container in the refrigerator for up to 36 hours.

Hemp Milk

Hemp is a great low-fat, lower-calorie source of protein. For flavoring, choose cinnamon or orange zest, based on your personal preference. On its own, hemp doesn't have a lot of taste. **MAKES 16 OUNCES**

> **$^1/_2$ cup hemp seeds**
> **1 tablespoon raw agave, or 2 Medjool dates, pitted**
> **$^1/_2$ teaspoon vanilla extract**
> **$^1/_2$ teaspoon cinnamon or orange zest**

Combine all of the ingredients in a high-speed blender and blend until smooth. Store in an airtight glass container in the refrigerator for up to 36 hours.

BREAKFAST

You've heard it before, but breakfast really is the most important meal of the day. You are fasting while you sleep; when you get out of bed, you need to wake up your metabolism and digestive system to start burning fat and creating energy. Drinking a smoothie or a juice first thing in the morning is great, but on those days when you want something more substantial, a protein or whole grain dish made the night before will get you out the door fast and well fed.

Roasted Vegetable Frittata

This is an easy-to-make, protein-rich dish that can be served hot, cold, or at room temperature. Make it the night before you want to serve it and reheat for breakfast, or pair it with a salad for a light lunch. **SERVES 2**

> 2 organic eggs
> 4 organic egg whites
> 1 cup Roasted Garden Vegetables (page 209)

Preheat the oven to 350°F. Coat an 8-inch round cake pan with cooking spray. In a medium bowl, whisk together the whole eggs and egg whites. Stir the roasted vegetables into the egg mixture. Pour the batter into the prepared cake pan. Bake uncovered for 45 minutes, until the batter is firm and just starting to brown on top. To reheat, place the frittata in a microwave for 45 to 60 seconds or warm in a 350°F oven for 15 minutes, covered with foil. Store covered and refrigerated for up to 5 days.

Steel-Cut Oatmeal

Steel-cut oats take a little longer to cook than rolled oats, but that's not a problem if you plan ahead. It can be served warm or at room temperature. **SERVES 4**

> 1 cup steel-cut oats
> Salt

Fill a 2-quart saucepan with 3 cups of water and set over medium heat. Add the oatmeal and salt to taste. Bring to a rolling boil. Turn off the heat, cover the pan, and leave on the stove for at least 30 minutes. Stir well and serve. Cover and refrigerate the leftovers. To reheat, warm in a saucepan on the stove over medium-low heat, stirring frequently, for about 5 minutes.

LUNCH

The lunch recipes are all easy to prepare ahead of time, take with you, and assemble before eating or serving. Plan ahead so you can bring your lunch with you. This will make eating healthier foods much easier for you.

Turkey Patty

With a little seasoning, a turkey patty has flavor to rival the best beef burger, with half the fat and calories. Serve warm, cold, or at room temperature. **SERVES 4**

> 1 pound ground turkey breast
> $1/4$ teaspoon garlic powder
> $1/4$ teaspoon cumin
> 1 teaspoon chopped parsley

In a bowl and using your hands to mix, combine the turkey, spices, and parsley. Shape into 4 patties. Spray a skillet with cooking spray and place over medium-high heat. Cook the patties for 6 minutes on each side. Store covered in the refrigerator for up to 5 days. To reheat, warm the patties in a microwave for 45 seconds, or heat in a sauté pan over medium heat for 4 minutes.

Tomato-Avocado Salad

This simple combination of tomatoes, nuts, and avocado is satisfying and delicious. A simple vinaigrette complements the flavor of the almonds. **SERVES 4**

> 1 pint cherry tomatoes
> 1 whole avocado, sliced
> 4 ounces Marcona almonds

¹⁄₄ cup Champagne Vinaigrette (page 230)

Slice the tomatoes in half. Arrange the tomatoes and avocado on a serving plate, or on 4 individual plates. Sprinkle with the almonds and drizzle with the vinaigrette. Serve immediately.

Spinach Salad

Spinach and strawberries keep this salad nutritious and flavorful.
SERVES 2 TO 4

2 handfuls baby spinach (about 2 cups)
¹⁄₂ cup sliced strawberries
¹⁄₂ cup shredded carrots
¹⁄₂ cup sliced cucumber
¹⁄₄ cup Balsamic Vinaigrette (page 212)

Place the spinach, strawberries, carrots, and cucumber in a medium bowl and toss with the vinaigrette. Serve immediately. If you're taking the salad to work, keep the vinaigrette in a separate container and toss just prior to eating.

Tomato-Fennel Salad

The crunchy fennel and sweet tomatoes combine to create a salad that is satisfying any time of year but especially on hot summer days or nights. **SERVES 6 TO 8**

1¹⁄₂ pounds heirloom tomatoes
1 small fennel bulb
2 tablespoons cold-pressed olive oil
2 tablespoons freshly squeezed lemon juice
1 tablespoon apple cider vinegar

continued >

Tomato-Fennel Salad, continued

> 1 teaspoon sea salt
> $^1/_2$ teaspoon freshly ground black pepper

Core and seed the tomatoes and cut into wedges. Remove the top of the fennel, saving some fronds for garnish. Slice the bulb thinly. Place the tomatoes and fennel in a medium bowl with all of the other ingredients and toss. Garnish with chopped fennel fronds. Serve immediately.

Roasted Veggie and Chicken Salad

Adding leftover sliced roasted chicken breast and roasted vegetables to a bed of mixed greens makes a quick and delicious meal. Serve chilled or at room temperature. **SERVES 2**

> 2 cups Roasted Root Vegetables with Butternut Squash (page 207)
>   or Roasted Garden Vegetables (page 209)
> 2 cups mixed greens
> 10 ounces Roasted Chicken Breast (page 196), sliced
> 4 tablespoons Lemon Vinaigrette (page 212)

Place all of the ingredients in a medium bowl, toss, and serve.

The undressed salad can be stored in an airtight container in the refrigerator for up to 2 days. If you're taking the salad to work with you, bring 2 tablespoons of vinaigrette in a separate container and toss right before eating.

Mediterranean Salad

Olives and feta cheese turn an ordinary salad into a Mediterranean specialty. Serve chilled or at room temperature. **SERVES 2**

> 8 ounces mixed greens
> 1 cucumber, chopped

12 cherry tomatoes, halved
1 cup cooked garbanzo beans, drained
$^{1}/_{2}$ cup black or kalamata olives, whole
2 ounces crumbled low-fat feta (optional)
4 tablespoons Lemon Vinaigrette (page 212)

Place all of the ingredients in a medium bowl, toss, and serve.

The undressed salad can be stored in an airtight container in the refrigerator for up to 2 days. If you're taking the salad to work with you, bring 2 tablespoons of vinaigrette in a separate container and toss right before eating.

Simple Kale Salad

The beauty of kale is that it doesn't get soggy in a salad, even if you add the dressing ahead of time. Serve chilled or at room temperature.
SERVES 2

2 cups chopped kale
$^{1}/_{4}$ cup sunflower seeds
$^{1}/_{2}$ cup shredded purple cabbage
$^{1}/_{2}$ cup shredded carrot
$^{1}/_{4}$ cup Curry Vinaigrette (page 213)

Place all of the ingredients in a medium bowl, toss, and serve. Can be made ahead of time and stored in the refrigerator for up to 24 hours.

Kale-Quinoa Salad

This salad is immensely satisfying with its combo of kale, strawberries, and quinoa. The Curry Vinaigrette (page 213) adds a sweet flavor that will convince even the biggest kale skeptic. Serve chilled or at room temperature. **SERVES 2**

continued >

Kale-Quinoa Salad, continued

>   2 handfuls chopped kale
>   ¹/₂ cup sliced strawberries
>   ¹/₂ cup Cooked Quinoa (page 206)
>   ¹/₄ cup sliced white onion
>   ¹/₄ cup Curry Vinaigrette (page 213)

Place all of the ingredients in a medium bowl, toss, and serve. Can be made ahead of time and stored in the refrigerator for up to 2 days.

Mixed Green Salad

This simple salad can be whipped up in a minute, which makes it easy to add greens to any meal. All of the vinaigrettes in the Dressings section (pages 211 to 214) go well with this salad, so choose according to your taste. **SERVES 4**

>   1 cup mixed greens
>   1 cup shredded carrots
>   1 medium cucumber, sliced
>   ¹/₄ cup vinaigrette (pages 211–214)

Place all of the ingredients in a medium bowl, toss, and serve.

The undressed salad can be stored in an airtight container in the refrigerator for up to 2 days. If you're taking the salad to work with you, bring 2 tablespoons of vinaigrette in a separate container and toss right before eating.

Heirloom Tomato Salad

Buy heirloom tomatoes in a multitude of colors for this dish that looks as beautiful as it tastes. **SERVES 4 AS A SIDE DISH OR 2 AS A MAIN DISH**

8 ounces green beans, cut into bite-size pieces
1 pound heirloom tomatoes, cut into bite-size pieces
1 small red onion, sliced
$^1/_2$ cup chopped walnuts
$^1/_4$ cup Balsamic Vinaigrette (page 212)
$^1/_4$ cup fresh basil leaves, sliced into ribbons, for garnish

Combine the beans, tomatoes, onion, and walnuts in a medium bowl and toss with the vinaigrette. Garnish with the basil ribbons. Serve immediately. Do not store in the refrigerator, as refrigeration will affect the flavor and texture of the heirloom tomatoes.

Fermented Veggies

Fermented vegetables make a delicious and digestion-enhancing side dish or snack. This recipe will last up to 6 months in your fridge, so double or triple the recipe and enjoy when you wish. You'll need a 32-ounce mason jar and a heavy rock (about the size of a golf ball) for the fermentation process. **MAKES ABOUT 24 OUNCES OF VEGGIES**

$^1/_2$ head red or green cabbage
2 carrots
1 stalk celery
1 (2-inch) piece ginger root, peeled
2 small cucumbers, peeled and seeded
1 small onion
1 small yellow bell pepper
1 clove garlic
3 tablespoons sea salt

Set aside two large cabbage leaves. Finely chop or shred all of the remaining vegetables and place in a large bowl, mixing them well. Massage the salt into the vegetables thoroughly, for at least 2 minutes. Place the salted vegetable mixture in a 32-ounce mason jar, leaving about 1 inch of space at the top to allow for expansion. Push the

continued >

Fermented Veggies, continued

mixture down, compressing it as much as possible. Add water to cover the vegetables. Lay the cabbage leaves on top of the chopped mixture and place the rock on top of the cabbage before sealing the jar. Store the jar in a dark cupboard. Open the jar once each day to release the pressure. It'll take approximately 4 days for the vegetables to ferment.

When it comes to determining whether or not you have successfully fermented your veggies, your nose will know. The veggies should smell sour, not rotten. If you have ever tasted or smelled sauerkraut, you will surely know the difference. Once they are fermented, you may remove the rock and store the sealed container of veggies in your fridge for up to 6 months.

Chicken Salad

This is a lighter version of chicken salad, made with Greek yogurt rather than mayonnaise. This boosts the flavor and protein, while reducing fat and calories. It's a great way to use up leftover chicken. Serve on a bed of lettuce or on bread as a sandwich. **SERVES 2**

> 1 Granny Smith apple, peeled and diced
> 2 cups shredded Roasted Chicken (page 194)
> ½ cup Greek yogurt
> 2 tablespoons Lemon Vinaigrette (page 212)
> ¼ cup grated parmesan (optional)

Combine all the ingredients in a medium bowl, stir well to mix, and serve. The salad can be stored in an airtight container in the refrigerator for up to 5 days.

Cucumber Salad

This salad can be served as a first course or a side dish. The longer it marinates, the better, so it's a great dish to make the day before. Serve cold or at room temperature. **SERVES 4**

2 cucumbers, peeled, seeded, and thinly sliced
1 white onion, thinly sliced
¹/₂ cup apple cider vinegar
Juice from ¹/₂ lemon
2 tablespoons organic raw honey
1 teaspoon red pepper flakes
Himalayan salt and pepper

Combine the cucumbers, onion, vinegar, ½ cup water, lemon juice, honey, and red pepper flakes in a medium bowl and mix well. Add salt and pepper to taste. Cover the bowl and place the salad in the refrigerator to marinate for at least 6 hours.

The salad can be stored, covered, in the refrigerator for up to 3 days.

SNACKS

When you hear the word *snack*, it may bring unhealthy thoughts of chips and munchies. In fact, a healthy combination of protein and carbohydrates will keep you satiated and fueled between meals. A healthy snack will keep you energized and keep your metabolism moving. When you're on the go, be sure to pack your snack and take it with you so you're never caught hungry without a healthy option.

Hummus

To avoid the preservatives often found in store-bought hummus, blend up your own with this fast and easy recipe. To bump up the flavor, add your choice of roasted red pepper, kalamata olives, or paprika. Serve chilled or at room temperature. MAKES 2 CUPS

1 (16-ounce) can garbanzo beans
1 clove garlic, peeled and chopped
2 teaspoons ground cumin

continued >

Hummus, continued

> $^1/_2$ teaspoon sea salt
> 1 tablespoon extra virgin olive oil
> 1 roasted red pepper, chopped (optional)
> $^1/_2$ cup chopped kalamata olives (optional)
> 1 teaspoon paprika (optional)

Rinse and drain the garbanzo beans, reserving the liquid. Combine the beans, garlic, cumin, salt, and olive oil in a food processor or blender. Blend on low speed, gradually adding the bean liquid, until a smooth consistency is achieved. Stir in the red pepper, olives, and paprika, and serve.

Store in the refrigerator for up to 14 days.

Hard-Boiled Eggs Filled with Smashed Avocado

Reduce the cholesterol and calories of a deviled egg by tossing the yolks and stuffing with avocado instead. **SERVES 2 TO 4**

> 4 large organic eggs
> Sea salt
> 1 avocado
> 1 lemon
> Freshly ground black pepper

Place the eggs in a 2-quart pot and cover completely with cold water. Add a pinch of salt to make the eggs easier to peel after cooking. Cover the pot and set it over high heat to boil. As soon as the water starts to boil, turn off the heat, and let the pot sit on the burner for 10 to 15 minutes. To see if the eggs are ready, whirl an egg on the counter. If it spins, it is done. If it turns slowly, put it back in the pan for another 5 minutes.

When the eggs are done, place them in a bowl of ice water to stop the cooking. When the eggs are cool enough to handle, peel them and slice each one lengthwise; set aside. Scoop out the yolk and discard. Mash the avocado with a fork. Add a squeeze of lemon juice and season to taste with salt and pepper. Fill each egg to overflowing with the avocado mixture, approximately 1½ tablespoons. The hard-boiled eggs can be made ahead, peeled, and kept refrigerated for up to 5 days. Mash the avocado and fill no more than a few hours before serving.

Chia Seed Pudding

This is the easiest pudding you'll ever make, and probably the healthiest. Chia seeds expedite weight loss and improve digestion, and when placed in liquid for a few hours, become thick and gelatinous, making a perfect pudding base. Serve chilled. **SERVES 2**

1 cup Almond Milk (page 181)
1 cup chia seeds

Combine the almond milk and chia seeds in a small bowl and mix well. Cover the bowl and place it in the refrigerator overnight or for up to 3 days.

Almond Butter

Store-bought nut butters typically include salt, sugar, and sometimes added oils. By making your own, you can ensure you get nothing but the nutrients of the almonds. **MAKES 1 CUP**

1 cup raw almonds

Blend the almonds in a blender or food processor until the nuts release their oil and the mixture becomes creamy, 5 to 10 minutes. Can be stored in an airtight container in a cool dry place or in the refrigerator for up to 2 months. The oils may separate over time, so mix well before using.

Ritual Trail Mix

This is our version of a trail mix. Raw nuts and dried berries keep it delicious and healthy. A little cacao will satisfy any chocolate craving.
SERVES 4

> ½ cup raw almonds
> ½ cup raw walnuts
> ½ cup unsweetened dried cranberries or mulberries
> ½ cup raw cacao nibs

Combine all of the ingredients in a medium bowl. Separate into ½-cup servings and store each in a resealable plastic bag in a cool dry place or the refrigerator for up to 1 month.

DINNER

We have saved the main entrées for dinner, as most of these will be served hot. As recommended earlier, if you cook your turkey and chicken once or twice a week and store it refrigerated, you can pull the cooked meat out as needed to save preparation time during the workweek.

Roasted Chicken

This is one of the simplest meals to prepare, and yet it seems fancy and indulgent. If you don't have 2 hours to spare for cooking the chicken, you can always pick up a couple of hot rotisserie chickens from the supermarket, or cook the chicken on your preparation day and store it until it's needed. Serve the roasted chicken warm, chilled, or at room temperature. **SERVES 4**

> 1 (5- to 6-pound) organic free-range roasting chicken
> Olive oil
> Garlic powder or salt-free spice blend
> 1 (14-ounce) can low-sodium chicken broth

Preheat the oven to 450°F. Rinse the chicken inside and out. Pat dry with paper towels. Rub the outside of the chicken with olive oil. Sprinkle with garlic powder. Place the chicken, breast side up, in a roasting pan in the oven. After 15 minutes, carefully pour the chicken broth over the chicken. Roast the chicken for another 2 hours, or until a meat thermometer inserted at the thigh reads 165°F. Baste every 15 minutes with the juices from the chicken. Remove from the oven and let rest for 15 minutes before carving.

If you are making the chicken for use later in the week, let it cool for about 30 minutes before placing it in the refrigerator, covered. The chicken can be stored in the refrigerator for up to 5 days. To reheat the chicken, warm it in a microwave for 2 minutes, or heat it in a 400°F oven for 15 minutes.

Butter Lettuce Tacos

We use butter lettuce in place of taco shells in this recipe to reduce calories and fat, and get more veggies in our diet. SERVES 4

> 1 head butter lettuce, washed and dried
> 1 pound ground turkey, cooked, or 1 pound shredded Roasted Chicken (page 194)
> 2 avocados, pitted and sliced
> 1 (3-ounce) container pico de gallo, or make your own by mixing diced plum tomatoes, white onions, and cilantro
> Shredded low-fat cheese (optional)
> Hot sauce (optional)

Use the 12 large outer leaves of butter lettuce as "taco shells" and shred the remaining lettuce. Fill each with 1 ounce turkey or chicken. Top with the shredded lettuce, avocado, pico de gallo, cheese, and hot sauce. Serve immediately. Store leftover turkey in the refrigerator for up to 5 days.

Variation: For a vegetarian option, replace the turkey with 1 (14.5-ounce) can rinsed and drained black beans.

Roasted Chicken Breast

Roasting chicken breasts in the oven allows you to make moist, perfectly cooked chicken every time. Pan-sear them first, to get that nice caramelized flavor and color. Serve warm, chilled, or at room temperature. **SERVES 4**

> 4 boneless, skinless organic chicken breasts
> Salt-free seasoning mix
> Cooking spray, either olive oil or coconut oil

Preheat the oven to 400°F. Season both sides of the chicken breasts. Spray a large ovenproof skillet with cooking spray and set over high heat. Place the chicken breasts in the pan and sauté until brown, about 3 minutes per side. Place the skillet in the oven and roast for 18 minutes. Remove the pan from the oven and let sit for at least 5 minutes before slicing. Store the chicken in the refrigerator for up to 5 days. To reheat, warm in a microwave for 45 seconds or in a 400°F oven for 15 minutes.

Ground Turkey

Cook up a package of ground turkey to use for filling the Butter Lettuce Tacos (page 195), Turkey-Stuffed Peppers (page 197), or in the Marinara Sauce (page 200). **SERVES 4**

> 1 pound ground turkey breast
> Salt-free seasoning blend

In a large skillet over medium-high heat, cook the turkey until the meat is no longer pink, about 7 minutes, breaking it up with a wooden spoon as it cooks. Season to taste several times throughout cooking. To reheat the turkey, warm it in a microwave for 45 seconds, or in a skillet over medium heat for 5 minutes. Store, covered, in the refrigerator for up to 5 days.

Turkey-Stuffed Peppers

This recipe skinnies up an Italian favorite. By using lean ground turkey breast, brown rice, and black beans, you keep all the flavor of the classic at a fraction of the calories and fat. SERVES 4

4 green bell peppers
1 cup cooked brown rice
2 cups cooked Ground Turkey (page 196)
1 (14-ounce) can unsalted tomato sauce
1 cup canned black beans, rinsed and drained
1 tablespoon chili powder
1 teaspoon garlic salt
Hot pepper sauce (optional)
¼ cup shredded low-fat cheese (optional)

Preheat the oven to 350°F. Cut the peppers in half lengthwise and remove the core and seeds. Place the peppers in a large saucepan and cover with water. Bring the water to a boil over high heat, cover, and boil for 3 minutes. Remove the saucepan from the heat and remove the peppers from the pan. Wipe the peppers dry and place them cut-side up in an 8-inch square baking dish.

In a medium bowl, combine the rice, turkey, tomato sauce, beans, chili powder, and garlic salt and mix well. Add hot sauce to taste. Generously stuff each pepper half with the turkey mixture. Cover the baking dish with foil. Bake for 25 minutes. Uncover, sprinkle with cheese, and bake for an additional 5 minutes. Serve hot.

To reheat, warm in a microwave for 2 minutes, or in a 350°F oven, covered with aluminum foil, for 15 minutes. Store leftovers in the refrigerator for up to 5 days.

Variation: For a vegetarian option, replace the turkey with 2 chopped Roasted Portobello Mushrooms (page 198).

Roasted Portobello Mushrooms

Portobello mushrooms have an almost meaty texture, and can be very satisfying in place of meat. You can slice them and add to a salad, put on a bun to eat in place of a burger, or chop and add anywhere you would normally use ground meat or poultry. Serve warm, chilled, or at room temperature. **SERVES 4**

4 large portobello mushrooms
4 tablespoons olive oil
1 teaspoon sea salt
1 tablespoon freshly ground black pepper

Preheat the oven to 425°F. Wash the mushrooms and remove the stems and gills. Toss the mushrooms with the oil, salt, and pepper in a medium bowl. Place in a single layer on an ungreased cookie sheet and roast for 15 to 20 minutes, until tender. Store, covered, in the refrigerator for up to 4 days. To reheat, warm in a microwave for 45 seconds, or in a skillet over medium heat for 5 minutes.

Fish Baked in Foil

By cooking fish in foil, you avoid both the smell that can permeate your home when you cook fish and a messy cleanup. Choose a sustainable white fish like Atlantic cod, Pacific halibut, or barramundi. **SERVES 2**

2 (6-ounce) fillets cod, halibut, or barramundi
¼ cup Lemon Vinaigrette (page 212)
1 red bell pepper, thinly sliced
½ cup shredded carrots
1 small summer squash, thinly sliced

Preheat the oven to 400°F. Set each fillet on a square piece of foil and rub with 1 tablespoon vinaigrette. Top each fillet with one-half of the

peppers, carrots, and squash and then drizzle with an additional tablespoon of vinaigrette. Cover each fillet with the foil, folding up and sealing all sides. Place on a baking sheet and bake for 20 to 25 minutes, until
the fish flakes easily with a fork. Serve immediately, but take care when
opening the packets not to burn yourself as there will be a lot of steam.

The cooked fish can be stored, covered, in the refrigerator for up to
3 days. To reheat, warm in a microwave for 90 seconds, or place
the cooked fish on a baking sheet and heat in a 375°F oven for 5 to
7 minutes.

Broiled Salmon

Salmon is a great addition to your diet due to its high omega-3 fatty
acid, protein, and amino acid content. Its meaty texture appeals to
many people who don't normally enjoy fish. It tastes great warm or
cold, so serve it for dinner and take leftovers for lunch later in the
week. **SERVES 2**

2 (6-ounce) salmon fillets
4 tablespoons Lemon-Dijon Vinaigrette (page 212)

Preheat the broiler. Line a rimmed baking sheet with foil and spray the
foil with nonstick cooking spray. Rub the salmon fillets with the vinaigrette and arrange them on the baking sheet. Broil the fillets until they
are just cooked through and golden brown, about 7 minutes. Do not
turn the fillets. Serve immediately.

The fillets can be stored, covered, in the refrigerator for up to 3 days. To
reheat, warm the fillets in a microwave for 90 seconds, or place the cooked
fish on a baking sheet and heat in a 375°F oven for 5 to 7 minutes.

Marinara Sauce

Serve this homemade sauce over cooked pasta or spaghetti squash (page 202). **SERVES 2 TO 4**

1 tablespoon olive oil
1 small onion, chopped
1 cup diced mixed veggies, such as carrots and bell peppers
1 (14.5-ounce) can diced tomatoes
1 (14.5-ounce) can unsalted tomato sauce
3 tablespoons tomato paste
1 tablespoon each chopped fresh basil, rosemary, and oregano,
  or 1 tablespoon dried Italian seasoning blend

Heat the olive oil in a large saucepan over medium heat. Add the onion and vegetables and cook, stirring frequently, until the onion is translucent, 5 to 7 minutes. Add the tomatoes, tomato sauce, tomato paste, and herbs. Simmer, uncovered, for 30 minutes, stirring frequently. Serve warm.

The sauce can be stored in an airtight container in the refrigerator for up to 7 days. To reheat, warm in a microwave for 1 minute or in a saucepan over medium heat for 5 minutes, or until heated through.

Pan-Seared Scallops

Scallops are a great source of vitamin B_{12} and omega-3 fatty acids. They have a sweet mild flavor that is delicious on its own. Just a little sea salt and pepper are all that you need to bring out the flavor. And best of all, they cook up in just minutes. **SERVES 4**

Olive oil
12 large sea scallops (about 1½ pounds)
½ teaspoon sea salt
½ teaspoon freshly ground black pepper

Gently rub olive oil over both sides of the scallops and then season both sides with salt and pepper. Heat a large skillet over high heat. Place the scallops in the skillet and sauté until browned on each side, about 2 minutes per side. Set on paper towels to soak up the excess liquid. Serve immediately.

Veggie Stir-Fry with Brown Rice

When you're short on time, stir-frying allows you to make a tasty meal in minutes. If your local market sells chopped vegetables, it reduces prep time even more. Feel free to substitute your choice of vegetables for any of those listed below. SERVES 4

    1 tablespoon coconut oil or sesame oil
    2 cups chopped broccoli
    1 medium red bell pepper, chopped
    1 medium yellow bell pepper, chopped
    1 cup chopped cauliflower
    ½ cup chopped celery
    4 heads baby bok choy, chopped
    1 (1-inch) piece fresh ginger root, peeled and grated
    1 tablespoon peeled and grated fresh garlic
    1 tablespoon Bragg Liquid Aminos
    2 cups cooked Brown Rice (page 207)

Heat a large skillet over medium-high heat. Add the oil and heat for 30 seconds, swirling to cover the pan. Add the broccoli, peppers, cauliflower, celery, and bok choy and stir-fry for 4 to 5 minutes, until the vegetables are cooked but still firm. Add the ginger, garlic, liquid aminos, and ¼ cup water and simmer until all the ingredients are tender. To serve, place one-quarter of the veggies on a bed of ½ cup cooked brown rice.

continued >

Veggie Stir-Fry with Brown Rice, continued

The stir-fry and rice can be stored, covered, in the refrigerator for up to 3 days. To reheat, warm in a microwave for 90 seconds or in saucepan over medium heat for 5 minutes, or until heated through.

Variation: For those nights when you want more than veggies, add shrimp for a protein-filled variation. Follow the instructions above, but add 1 pound of peeled and deveined shrimp along with the ginger, garlic, liquid aminos, and water. Cook until the shrimp turns pink, about 3 or 4 minutes.

Spaghetti Squash with Turkey Marinara Sauce

Spaghetti squash is a unique squash whose flesh separates into spaghetti-like strands when it's cooked. It can be used in place of spaghetti in nearly any recipe. It has a sweet flavor that blends particularly well with this marinara sauce. SERVES 4

1 spaghetti squash
2 cups Marinara Sauce (page 200)
1 cup cooked Ground Turkey (page 196)

Preheat the oven to 400°F. Place the whole squash on an ungreased baking sheet and bake for 1 hour. Cut the squash open at the equator (not lengthwise), carefully remove the seeds and pulp, and separate the strands with a fork.

In a large saucepan over medium heat, combine the marinara sauce and ground turkey. Cook until warmed through, about 5 minutes. To serve, separate the spaghetti squash into 4 portions, making a nest on each plate. Cover each with ½ cup of the marinara-turkey sauce.

The squash can be stored, covered, in the refrigerator for up to 5 days. To reheat, warm in a microwave for 2 minutes or in a saucepan over medium heat until heated through, about 10 minutes.

Variation: For a vegetarian option, omit the ground turkey.

Thai Coconut Curry

If you've tried tofu but can't get over the fact that it has no flavor, this dish is for you. The creamy coconut milk, onion, peppers, and curry make an exotic flavor combination that the tofu soaks up wonderfully. This can be served warm, chilled, or at room temperature. **SERVES 2**

2 cups light coconut milk
4 ounces Thai curry paste
1 (16-ounce) block firm organic tofu
1 red bell pepper, thinly sliced
1 yellow bell pepper, thinly sliced
1 small white onion, thinly sliced
1 cup broccoli florets

In a small bowl, combine the coconut milk and curry paste until well blended. Slice the tofu into bite-size chunks. Place the tofu, peppers, onion, and broccoli in a wok and pour the coconut-curry mixture over the top. Cook over medium-high heat for about 10 minutes, until all the ingredients are warmed through. Serve immediately.

The curry can be stored, covered, in the refrigerator for up to 5 days. To reheat, warm in a microwave for 90 seconds, stirring after 45 seconds, or in saucepan over medium heat for 10 minutes.

SOUPS

Soups are an easy way to incorporate more veggies into your diet. Canned soups, unfortunately, are generally full of sodium, preservatives, and extra calories. By making your own, you can keep them healthy.

Tomato-Vegetable Soup

Soup can be a delicious appetizer or a satisfying meal. Making soup from scratch allows you to control the salt and fat, making it much healthier than the canned alternative. **SERVES 2 TO 4**

> 4 cups canned vegetable broth
> 3 cups chopped fresh vegetables (such as celery, carrots, peas, corn, green beans, cauliflower, and broccoli), or 1 (16-ounce) bag frozen chopped vegetables
> 1 (14.5-ounce) can diced tomatoes
> Freshly ground black pepper
> Garlic powder
> Red pepper flakes (optional)

In a large stockpot, combine the broth, 1 cup water, the vegetables, and tomatoes. Season to taste with the pepper, garlic powder, and red pepper flakes. Bring to a boil, reduce the heat, and simmer for 20 to 30 minutes, until all of the vegetables are tender. Serve warm. Store, covered, in the refrigerator for up to 7 days. To reheat, warm in a microwave for 90 seconds, stirring after 45 seconds, or in a saucepan over medium heat for 5 minutes, or until heated through.

Carrot-Ginger Soup

The zing of ginger balances the sweetness of the carrots in this delicious, easy-to-make soup. A touch of rice thickens it without any dairy. **SERVES 2 TO 4**

> 2 shallots, sliced
> 1 tablespoon olive oil
> 2 cups chopped carrots
> 1 (1-inch) piece ginger root, peeled and grated
> 1 tablespoon white or brown rice
> 2 cups canned vegetable broth
> Sea salt and freshly ground black pepper

In a large saucepan over medium heat, sauté the shallots in the olive oil until translucent. Add the carrots, ginger, rice, broth, and 3 cups water. Simmer until the carrots and rice are tender, about 15 minutes. Puree the ingredients in the pot using a handheld immersion blender, or transfer the soup to a blender to puree, in batches if necessary. Add salt and pepper to taste. Serve warm or at room temperature.

The soup can be stored in the refrigerator for up to 7 days. To reheat, warm in a microwave for 90 seconds, stirring after 45 seconds, or in a saucepan over medium heat for 5 minutes, or until heated through.

Curried Raw Cream of Carrot Soup

Avocado adds a satisfying nondairy creaminess to this soup of curried carrots. Note: If you don't have a high-speed blender, you may need to juice the carrots first. **SERVES 2 TO 4**

1 pound carrots
$1/2$ avocado
Juice of 1 lime
$3/4$ teaspoon curry powder
$1/4$ teaspoon Himalayan sea salt
A few springs cilantro, for garnish
1 tablespoon chopped unsalted cashews, for garnish

Combine the carrots (or carrot juice; see headnote), avocado, lime juice, curry powder, and salt in a high-speed blender and blend until smooth. Pour into bowls and garnish with cilantro and chopped cashews. Serve at room temperature. Leftovers can be stored, covered, in the refrigerator for up to 3 days.

Raw Red Pepper Soup

We use raw cashews in place of dairy to add creaminess and protein to this sweet red pepper soup. **SERVES 2**

> 2 red bell peppers, diced
> $^1/_3$ cup raw cashews
> $^1/_2$ teaspoon sea salt
> 1 small clove garlic, peeled and chopped
> A pinch of cayenne pepper (optional)
> A pinch of red pepper flakes (optional)

Combine the peppers, cashews, salt, garlic, and cayenne in a high-speed blender and blend until smooth. Pour into bowls and garnish with red pepper flakes. Serve at room temperature. Leftovers can be stored, covered, in the refrigerator for up to 3 days.

SIDES

These side dishes add some balance to your evening meal, or they can be used to complement your lunch salad.

Cooked Quinoa

Quinoa (pronounced keen-wah) is a grain that is high in fiber and protein. It can be used in place of rice to increase the nutrition profile of any meal. Quinoa can be served warm, chilled, or at room temperature. **SERVES 4 (ABOUT 2 CUPS COOKED QUINOA)**

> 1 cup water or vegetable broth
> $^1/_2$ cup quinoa

In a small saucepan, bring the water to a boil over high heat. Add the quinoa to the boiling water, stir, and reduce the heat to low. Cover and simmer until tender, about 15 minutes. Remove from the heat and let sit for 5 minutes. Fluff with a fork before serving.

Leftovers can be stored, covered, in the refrigerator for up to 7 days. To reheat, warm in a microwave for 30 seconds or in a small saucepan over medium heat for 5 minutes, stirring frequently.

Brown Rice

Brown rice is the unrefined, unprocessed version of white rice, and is a better choice when it comes to your health. It is high in fiber and rich in protein, calcium, and magnesium. The rice can be served warm or at room temperature. **SERVES 4**

1 cup brown rice

In a medium saucepan over high heat, combine the rice with 2 cups water and heat until the water boils. Reduce the heat to medium-low and simmer for 20 minutes, or until all of the water is absorbed. Fluff the rice with a fork before serving.

Leftovers can be stored, covered, in the refrigerator for up to 7 days. To reheat, warm in a microwave for 30 seconds or in a small saucepan over medium heat for 5 minutes, stirring frequently.

Roasted Root Vegetables with Butternut Squash

Roasting root vegetables and squash brings out all of their natural sugars, leaving them sweet and caramelized. They can be eaten as a side, added to a salad, or blended with water or vegetable broth into a flavorful soup. **SERVES 4**

continued >

Roasted Root Vegetables with Butternut Squash, continued

 1 large sweet potato, peeled and chopped
 4 large carrots, peeled and sliced
 2 large beets, stems removed and chopped
 $1/2$ medium butternut squash, peeled and chopped
 2 tablespoons olive oil
 1 teaspoon sea salt or kosher salt
 $1/2$ teaspoon freshly cracked black pepper

Preheat the oven to 400°F. Place the vegetables in a medium bowl and toss with the olive oil; season with the salt and pepper. Roast in the oven for 30 to 40 minutes, tossing every 10 minutes, until cooked through. Serve warm, chilled, or at room temperature.

The vegetables can be stored, covered, in the refrigerator for up to 7 days. To reheat, warm in a microwave for 30 seconds, in the oven at 325°F for 10 minutes, or in a skillet over medium heat for 7 minutes, or until heated through.

Roasted Beets

Roasted beets are nature's candy. Once roasted, their natural sugars caramelize them, making them very sweet. They can be eaten as a side dish or added to a salad in place of fruit, especially in the winter when beets are much easier to find than fresh berries. Serve warm, chilled, or at room temperature. SERVES 4

 4 large or 8 small red, yellow, or orange beets

Preheat the oven to 400°F. Wash and stem the beets. (There's no need to peel them.) Wrap each beet individually in foil. Place the wrapped beets on a baking sheet and bake until the beets are tender enough to pierce easily with a knife, 40 to 50 minutes, depending on their size. Peel off the foil and set aside until cool enough to handle. You may want to wear gloves, as the beets may stain your hands for a good day or two otherwise.

Leftovers can be stored, covered, in the refrigerator for up to 7 days. To reheat, warm in a microwave for 30 seconds or in the oven at 325°F for 10 minutes.

Roasted Cauliflower

Although cauliflower is full of antioxidants, is loaded with fiber, and has anti-inflammatory properties, it can taste kind of boring. Not so when it is roasted. It becomes so tender and sweet that you will almost forget you are eating a vegetable! Serve warm, chilled, or at room temperature.
SERVES 4

> 1 head cauliflower (about 2 pounds)
> 2 tablespoons olive oil
> 1 teaspoon sea salt or kosher salt
> $1/2$ teaspoon freshly ground black pepper

Preheat the oven to 400°F. Cut the florets from the head, slicing the larger ones in half. Toss lightly in the oil, salt, and pepper. Roast in a 13 by 9-inch baking dish for 30 to 40 minutes, tossing every 10 minutes, until the cauliflower is tender and starting to brown.

Leftovers can be stored, covered, in the refrigerator for up to 7 days. To reheat, warm in a microwave for 30 seconds or in the oven at 325°F for 10 minutes.

Roasted Garden Vegetables

Just like root vegetables, garden vegetables are sweeter and tastier when they are roasted with a bit of olive oil and a pinch of sea salt. They make a great side dish or a flavorful addition to a chopped salad. Serve warm, chilled, or at room temperature. **SERVES 4**

continued >

Roasted Garden Vegetables, continued

1 red bell pepper, chopped

2 zucchini, chopped

2 large yellow squash, chopped

1 cup broccoli florets

2 tablespoons olive oil

1 teaspoon sea salt or kosher salt

$1/2$ teaspoon freshly ground black pepper

Preheat the oven to 400°F. Combine the chopped vegetables with the broccoli in a 13 by 9-inch baking dish. Toss lightly with the oil and season with the salt and pepper. Roast for 30 to 40 minutes, tossing every 10 minutes, until the vegetables are tender and starting to brown.

Leftovers can be stored, covered, in the refrigerator for up to 7 days. To reheat, warm in a microwave for 30 seconds or in the oven at 325°F for 10 minutes.

Roasted Asparagus

You don't need a grill to get that great charred flavor of roasted asparagus. These stalks are so naturally flavorful that you won't even miss the hollandaise sauce. Serve warm, chilled, or at room temperature.

SERVES 4

1 bunch asparagus spears

1 tablespoon olive oil

Sea salt or kosher salt

Freshly cracked black pepper

Preheat the oven to 400°F. Cut off the tough white bottom from each spear. In a bowl, toss the spears lightly in the oil and season to taste with the salt and pepper. Roast on a baking sheet for 10 to 15 minutes, tossing every 5 minutes, until tender.

Leftovers can be stored, covered, in the refrigerator for up to 7 days. To reheat, warm in a microwave for 30 seconds or in the oven at 325°F for 5 minutes.

Sautéed Spinach

If you haven't sautéed spinach before, you'll be surprised to see how much it wilts when cooked. Steaming spinach can leave it tasting bitter, while sautéing brings out its natural flavor. Do not overcook. Stop cooking when it's bright green and wilted. **SERVES 2**

> **1 pound baby spinach**
> **1 tablespoon salt-free seasoning, such as garlic powder, red pepper flakes, or multi-seasoning blend**

Spray a large skillet with cooking spray, and warm over high heat. Add the spinach and sprinkle with seasoning. Sauté until wilted, tossing constantly, about 2 minutes. Serve immediately.

Leftovers can be stored, covered, in the refrigerator for up to 3 days. To reheat, warm in a microwave for 30 seconds or in a sauté pan over medium heat for 2 minutes.

DRESSINGS

Homemade vinaigrettes can be made ahead of time and then stored in sealed containers for up to 2 weeks. You can also double or triple these recipes, so you'll have dressing on hand whenever you need it. All of our dressings are made with vinegar or lemon juice—both because they add delicious flavor to any salad and because they are believed to enable weight loss since they prolong the sensation of satiety after eating.

Lemon Vinaigrette

This light dressing isn't overpowering. The lemon helps enhance the natural flavors of vegetables. **MAKES ABOUT ⅓ CUP**

> Juice of 2 fresh lemons
> ¼ cup olive oil
> 1 teaspoon sea salt or kosher salt
> 1 teaspoon freshly ground black pepper

Whisk all ingredients together. Store, covered, in a cool, dark place for up to 2 weeks. Whisk before serving.

Lemon-Dijon Vinaigrette

A creamier version of the vinaigrette above. **MAKES ABOUT ½ CUP**

> Juice of 2 lemons
> 1 tablespoon Dijon mustard
> ¼ cup olive oil
> 1 teaspoon sea salt or kosher salt
> 1 teaspoon freshly ground black pepper

Whisk all ingredients together. Store, covered, in a cool, dark place for up to 2 weeks. Whisk before serving.

Balsamic Vinaigrette

Balsamic vinegar is made from just-harvested white grapes and is cooked, concentrated, and aged to produce a sweet flavor that can make any salad taste gourmet. **MAKES ABOUT ½ CUP**

> 2 tablespoons balsamic vinegar
> ¼ cup olive oil
> 1 teaspoon raw honey (optional)

1 teaspoon sea salt or kosher salt
1 teaspoon freshly ground black pepper

Whisk all ingredients together. Store, covered, in a cool, dark place for up to 2 weeks. Whisk before serving.

Champagne Vinaigrette

Champagne vinegar has a sweet, light flavor that is less intense than balsamic. It adds a citrusy note to any vinaigrette. MAKES ABOUT $1/2$ CUP

2 tablespoons champagne vinegar
$1/4$ cup olive oil
1 teaspoon sea salt or kosher salt
1 teaspoon freshly ground black pepper

Whisk all ingredients together. Store, covered, in a cool, dark place for up to 2 weeks. Whisk before serving.

Curry Vinaigrette

These ingredients perfectly complement any tough or bitter green, especially kale. The complexity of flavors in this vinaigrette will have your dinner guests asking for the recipe. MAKES ABOUT $1^{1}/_{2}$ CUPS

$1/4$ cup apple cider vinegar
$1/4$ cup freshly squeezed orange juice
$1/4$ cup rice vinegar
$1/2$ cup olive oil
1 tablespoon curry powder
1 teaspoon vanilla extract
1 teaspoon sea salt
1 teaspoon freshly cracked black pepper

Whisk all ingredients together. Store, covered, in a cool, dark place for up to 2 weeks. Whisk before serving.

Apple Cider Vinaigrette

Apple cider vinegar has great health benefits, since it's made from fermented apple cider. It balances the tamari nicely for a sweet, nutty-flavored dressing. **MAKES ABOUT 1 CUP**

- $^1/_2$ cup apple cider vinegar
- $^1/_3$ cup olive oil
- 1 teaspoon tamari
- 1 teaspoon raw honey or raw agave
- Sea salt or kosher salt
- Freshly cracked black pepper

Whisk the vinegar, oil, tamari, and honey together. Season to taste with salt and pepper. Store, covered, in a cool, dark place for up to 2 weeks. Whisk before serving.

ABOUT THE AUTHORS

Lori Kenyon Farley (right) and Marra St. Clair (left) are the founders of Southern California's popular Ritual Juice Cleanse program and considered among the top cleansing experts in the United States. Lori is a hedge-fund manager turned certified nutritional consultant, and Marra is a certified Pilates instructor, personal trainer, and nutritional consultant. Visit the Ritual website, www.ritualcleanse.com, for more information.

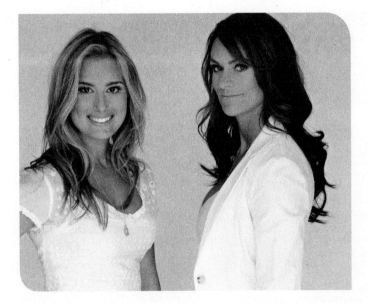

INDEX